PAIN MEDICINE
A CASE-BASED
LEARNING SERIES

The Knee

PAIN MEDICINE
A CASE-BASED
LEARNING SERIES

The Knee

STEVEN D. WALDMAN, MD, JD

ELSEVIER

Elsevier
1600 John F. Kennedy Blvd.
Ste 1800
Philadelphia, PA 19103-2899

PAIN MEDICINE: A CASE-BASED LEARNING SERIES   ISBN: 978-0-323-76258-8
THE KNEE

Notice

Library of Congress Control Number: 2021936715

Executive Content Strategist: Michael Houston
Content Development Specialist: Jeannine Carrado/Laura Klien
Director, Content Development: Ellen Wurm-Cutter
Publishing Services Manager: Shereen Jameel
Senior Project Manager: Karthikeyan Murthy
Design Direction: Amy Buxton

Printed in India

Last digit is the print number: 9 8 7 6 5 4 3 2

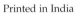
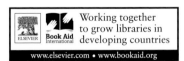

Working together
to grow libraries in
developing countries

www.elsevier.com • www.bookaid.org

"When you go after honey with a balloon, the great thing is to not let the bees know you're coming."

WINNIE THE POOH

It's Harder Than It Looks
MAKING THE CASE FOR CASE-BASED LEARNING

For sake of full disclosure, I was one of those guys. You know, the ones who wax poetic about how hard it is to teach our students how to do procedures. Let me tell you, teaching folks how to do epidurals on women in labor certainly takes its toll on the coronary arteries. It's true, I am amazing. . .I am great. . .I have nerves of steel. Yes, I could go on like this for hours. . .but you have heard it all before. But, it's again that time of year when our new students sit eagerly before us, full of hope and dreams. . .and that harsh reality comes slamming home. . .it is a lot harder to teach beginning medical students "doctoring" than it looks.

A few years ago, I was asked to teach first-year medical and physician assistant students how to take a history and perform a basic physical exam. In my mind I thought "this should be easy. . .no big deal". I won't have to do much more than show up. After all, I was the guy who wrote that amazing book on physical diagnosis. After all, I had been teaching medical students, residents, and fellows how to do highly technical (and dangerous, I might add) interventional pain management procedures since right after the Civil War. Seriously, it was no big deal...I could do it in my sleep. . .with one arm tied behind my back. . .blah. . .blah. . .blah.

For those of you who have had the privilege of teaching "doctoring," you already know what I am going to say next. *It's harder than it looks!* Let me repeat this to disabuse any of you who, like me, didn't get it the first time. *It is harder than it looks!* I only had to meet with my first-year medical and physician assistant students a couple of times to get it through my thick skull: **It really is harder than it looks**. In case you are wondering, the reason that our students look back at us with those blank, confused, bored, and ultimately dismissive looks is simple: They lack context. That's right, they lack the context to understand what we are talking about.

It's really that simple. . .or hard. . .depending on your point of view or stubbornness, as the case may be. To understand why context is king, you have to look only as far as something as basic as the Review of Systems. The Review of Systems is about as basic as it gets, yet why is it so perplexing to our students? Context. I guess it should come as no surprise to anyone that the student is completely lost when you talk about. . .let's say. . .the "constitutional" portion of the Review of Systems, without the context of what a specific constitutional finding, say a fever or chills, might mean to a patient who is suffering from the acute onset of headaches. If you tell the student that you need to ask about fever, chills, and the other "constitutional" stuff and you take it no further, you might as well be talking about the

International Space Station. Just save your breath; it makes absolutely no sense to your students. Yes, they want to please, so they will memorize the elements of the Review of Systems, but that is about as far as it goes. On the other hand, if you present the case of Jannette Patton, a 28-year-old first-year medical resident with a fever and headache, you can see the lights start to come on. By the way, this is what Jannette looks like, and as you can see, Jannette is sicker than a dog. This, at its most basic level, is what *Case-Based Learning* is all about.

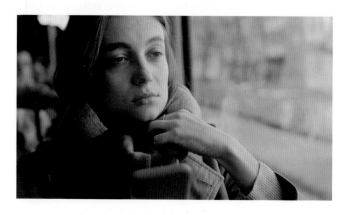

I would like to tell you that, smart guy that I am, I immediately saw the light and became a convert to *Case-Based Learning*. But truth be told, it was COVID-19 that really got me thinking about *Case-Based Learning*. Before the COVID-19 pandemic, I could just drag the students down to the med/surg wards and walk into a patient room and riff. Everyone was a winner. For the most part, the patients loved to play along and thought it was cool. The patient and the bedside was all I needed to provide the context that was necessary to illustrate what I was trying to teach—the why headache and fever don't mix kind of stuff. Had COVID-19 not rudely disrupted my ability to teach at the bedside, I suspect that you would not be reading this *Preface*, as I would not have had to write it. Within a very few days after the COVID-19 pandemic hit, my days of bedside teaching disappeared, but my students still needed context. This got me focused on how to provide the context they needed. The answer was, of course, *Case-Based Learning*. What started as a desire to provide context...because it really was **harder than it looked**...led me to begin work on this eight-volume *Case-Based Learning* textbook series. What you will find within these volumes are a bunch of fun, real-life cases that help make each patient come alive for the student. These cases provide the contextual teaching points that make it easy for the teacher to explain why, when Jannette's chief complaint is, *"My head is killing me and I've got a fever,"* it is a big deal.

Have fun!

Steven D. Waldman, MD, JD
Spring 2021

ACKNOWLEDGMENTS

A very special thanks to my editors, Michael Houston PhD, Jeannine Carrado, and Karthikeyan Murthy, for all of their hard work and perseverance in the face of disaster. Great editors such as Michael, Jeannine, and Karthikeyan make their authors look great, for they not only understand how to bring the Three Cs of great writing. . .Clarity + Consistency + Conciseness. . .to the author's work, but unlike me, they can actually punctuate and spell!

Steven D. Waldman, MD, JD

P.S. . . .Sorry for all the ellipses, guys!

CONTENTS

Rose Williams

A 72-Year-Old Female With Right Knee Pain

- Learn the common causes of knee pain.
- Develop an understanding of the unique anatomy of the knee joint.
- Develop an understanding of the causes of arthritis of the knee.
- Learn the clinical presentation of osteoarthritis of the knee.
- Learn how to use physical examination to identify pathology of the knee joint.
- Develop an understanding of the treatment options for osteoarthritis of the knee joint.
- Learn the appropriate testing options to help diagnose osteoarthritis of the knee joint.
- Learn to identify red flags in patients who present with knee pain.
- Develop an understanding of the role in interventional pain management in the treatment of knee pain.

Rose Williams

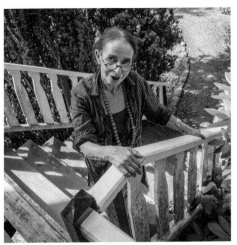

Rose Williams is a 72-year-old seamstress with the chief complaint of, "I can't walk up the stairs to my house because of my knee." Rose went on to say that she wouldn't have bothered me, but it was becoming harder and harder to make it up her front steps after coming home from work. Rose said that 50 years of pinning hems and cuffs had finally caught up with her. "Doc, I don't know what I would do if I didn't go to work every day, but the getting down on my knees and getting up again is getting harder and harder. The pain at work is bad enough, but the last few weeks, when I get home, I have to use my arms to help pull me up my front stairs."

I asked Rose if anything like this has happened before. She shook her head and said, "I'm in pretty good shape for 72 years old, but my right knee is giving me a fit. I have never been a sound sleeper, but this knee must wake me up 20 times a night. I have been using my heating pad, but you know I live alone and I am afraid to leave it on at night."

I asked Rose about any antecedent trauma to the right knee. She thought about it for a minute and said that she really couldn't remember any injuries, but she did tend to get down on her right knee when she was marking cuffs and hems.

I asked Rose to point with one finger to show me where it hurts the most. Rose didn't point, but instead cupped the front of her right knee in her palm and rubbed it, responding, "The whole knee hurts. Doc, the other thing is, sometimes I feel this grating sensation, especially when I first get up in the morning." She denied popping or catching with flexion and extension. I asked if she had any fever or chills and she shook her head no. "What about steroids?" I asked. "Did you ever take any cortisone or drugs like that?" Rose again shook her head no and said, "Doc, you know me. I'm a tough old bird and I wouldn't bother you if it didn't really hurt. I love my job—it's my life! But this knee has really got me worried. I have to be able to get into my house or what will become of me?"

On physical examination, Rose was afebrile. Her respirations were 18 and her pulse was 74 and regular. Her blood pressure (BP) was normal at

122/74. Her head, eyes, ears, nose, throat (HEENT) exam was normal, as was her cardiopulmonary examination. Her thyroid was normal. Her abdominal examination revealed no abnormal mass or organomegaly. There was no costovertebral angle (CVA) tenderness. There was no peripheral edema. Her low back examination was unremarkable. I did a rectal exam and pelvic, which were both normal. Visual inspection of the knee revealed no cutaneous lesions or obvious hernia or other abnormal mass. The area overlying the right knee was warm to touch. Palpation of the right knee revealed mild diffuse tenderness, with no obvious synovitis or point tenderness. On ballottement of the right knee, there was a suggestion of mild effusion. There was mild crepitus, but I did not appreciate any popping or catching. Range of motion was decreased, with pain exacerbated with active and passive range of motion. The left knee examination was normal, as was examination of her other major joints, other than some mild osteoarthritis in the fingers. A careful neurologic examination of the upper and lower extremities revealed there was no evidence of peripheral or entrapment neuropathy, and the deep tendon reflexes were normal.

Key Clinical Points—What's Important and What's Not

THE HISTORY

- No history of acute knee trauma
- No fever or chills
- Gradual onset of right knee pain over the last several weeks with exacerbation of pain with knee use
- Grating sensation in the right knee
- Sleep disturbance
- Difficulty walking up stairs due to pain
- Pain on kneeling

THE PHYSICAL EXAMINATION

- The patient is afebrile
- Normal visual inspection of knee
- Palpation of right knee reveals diffuse tenderness
- No point tenderness
- Mild warmth of right knee
- Crepitus and pain with range of motion
- No evidence of infection
- Suggestion of a mild effusion
- No active synovitis

OTHER FINDINGS OF NOTE

- Normal BP
- Normal HEENT examination
- Normal cardiovascular examination
- Normal pulmonary examination
- Normal abdominal examination
- No peripheral edema
- No groin mass or inguinal hernia
- No CVA tenderness
- Normal pelvic exam
- Normal rectal exam
- Normal upper extremity neurologic examination, motor and sensory examination
- Examination of joints other than the right knee were normal other than some mild osteoarthritis of the hands

 ## What Tests Would You Like to Order?

The following tests were ordered:
- Plain radiograph of the right knee

TEST RESULTS

The plain radiographs of the right knee revealed significant joint space narrowing and osteophyte formation consistent with severe osteoarthritis (Fig. 1.1).

 ## CLINICAL CORRELATION—PUTTING IT ALL TOGETHER

What is the diagnosis?
- Osteoarthritis of the right knee joint

The Science Behind the Diagnosis

ANATOMY OF THE KNEE JOINTS

Although both clinicians and laypeople think of the knee joint as a single joint, from the viewpoint of understanding the functional anatomy, it is more helpful to think of the knee as two separate but interrelated joints: the femoral-tibial joint and the femoral-patellar joint (Fig. 1.2). The two joints share a common synovial cavity, and dysfunction of one joint can easily affect the function of the other.

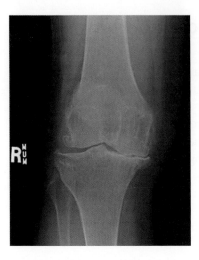

Fig. 1.1 Osteoarthritis of the knee. Anteroposterior standing knee X-ray with joint space loss, especially in the medial compartment and osteophytes bilaterally. (From Vincent TL, Watt FE. Osteoarthritis. *Medicine*. 2018:46[3]:187–195 [Fig. 3C].)

The femoral-tibial joint is made up of the articulation of the femur and the tibia. Interposed between the two bones are two fibrocartilaginous structures known as the medial and lateral menisci (Fig. 1.3). The menisci help transmit the forces placed on the femur across the joint onto the tibia. The menisci have the property of plasticity in that they are able to change their shape in response to the variable forces placed on the joint through its complex range of motion. The medial and lateral menisci are relatively avascular and receive the bulk of their nourishment from the synovial fluid, which means that there is little potential for healing when these important structures are traumatized.

The primary function of the femoral-patellar joint is to use the patella, which is a large sesamoid bone embedded in the quadriceps tendon, to improve the mechanical advantage of the quadriceps muscle. The medial and lateral articular surfaces of the sesamoid interface with the articular groove of the femur (Fig. 1.4). In extension, only the superior pole of the patella is in contact with the articular surface of the femur. As the knee flexes, the patella is drawn superiorly into the trochlear groove of the femur.

CLINICAL PRESENTATION OF ARTHRITIS OF THE KNEE JOINT

Arthritis of the knee is a common painful condition. The knee joint is susceptible to the development of arthritis from a variety of conditions that have the ability to damage the joint cartilage. Osteoarthritis is the most common form of arthritis that results in knee pain; rheumatoid arthritis and

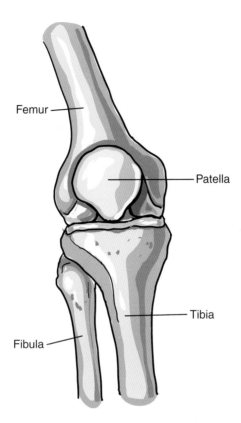

Fig. 1.2 Functional anatomy of the knee is easier to understand if it is viewed as two separate but interrelated joints: the femoral-tibial and the femoral-patellar joints. (From Waldman SD. *Physical Diagnosis of Pain: An Atlas of Signs and Symptoms*. 3rd ed. St Louis: Elsevier; 2016: Fig. 195.1.)

posttraumatic arthritis are also common causes of knee pain. Less common causes of arthritis-induced knee pain include collagen vascular diseases, infection, villonodular synovitis, and Lyme disease. Acute infectious arthritis is usually accompanied by significant systemic symptoms, including fever and malaise, and should be easily recognized; it is treated with culture and antibiotics rather than injection therapy. Collagen vascular disease generally presents as a polyarthropathy rather than a monoarthropathy limited to the knee joint, although knee pain secondary to collagen vascular disease responds exceedingly well to the treatment modalities described here.

SIGNS AND SYMPTOMS

The majority of patients with osteoarthritis or posttraumatic arthritis of the knee complain of pain localized around the knee and distal femur. Activity makes the pain worse, whereas rest and heat provide some relief.

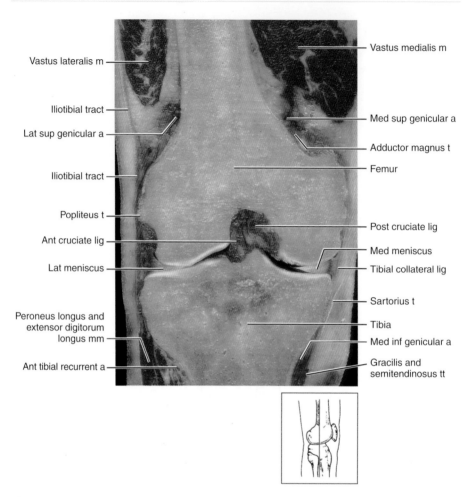

Vastus lateralis m

Iliotibial tract

Lat sup genicular a

Iliotibial tract

Popliteus t

Ant cruciate lig

Lat meniscus

Peroneus longus and extensor digitorum longus mm

Ant tibial recurrent a

Vastus medialis m

Med sup genicular a

Adductor magnus t

Femur

Post cruciate lig

Med meniscus

Tibial collateral lig

Sartorius t

Tibia

Med inf genicular a

Gracilis and semitendinosus tt

Fig. 1.3 Coronal view of the knee. *a*, artery; *t*, tendon; *n*, nerve; *lig*, ligament; *m*, muscle; *tt*, tendons. (From Kang HS, Ahn JM, Resnick D. *MRI of the Extremities*. Philadelphia: Saunders; 2002:301.)

The pain is constant and is characterized as aching in nature; it may interfere with sleep. Some patients complain of a grating or popping sensation with use of the joint, and crepitus may be present on physical examination.

In addition to pain, patients often experience a gradual reduction in functional ability because of decreasing knee range of motion, making simple everyday tasks such as walking, climbing stairs, and getting in and out of a car quite difficult (Fig. 1.5). With continued disuse, muscle wasting may occur, and a frozen knee due to adhesive capsulitis may develop.

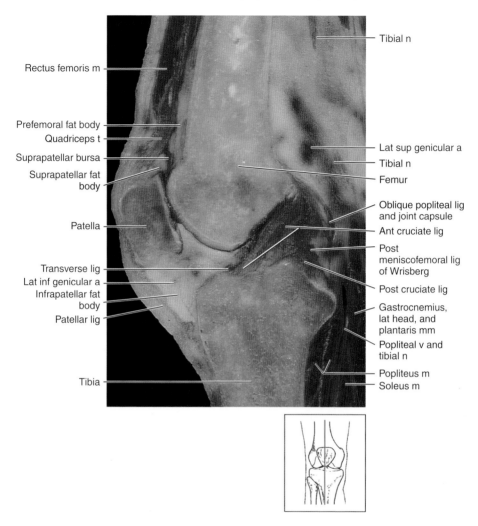

Fig. 1.4 Sagittal view of the knee. (From Kang HS, Ahn JM, Resnick D. *MRI of the Extremities*. Philadelphia: Saunders; 2002:341.)

TESTING

Plain radiography is indicated in all patients who present with knee pain (Fig. 1.6). Based on the patient's clinical presentation, additional testing may be warranted, including a complete blood count, erythrocyte sedimentation rate, and antinuclear antibody testing. Magnetic resonance (MRI) and ultrasound imaging of the knee is indicated if internal derangement, aseptic necrosis, or an occult mass or tumor is suspected, or if the diagnosis is in question (Figs. 1.7 and 1.8).

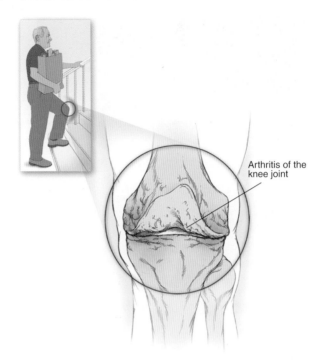

Fig. 1.5 Patients suffering from osteoarthritis of the knee often experience a gradual reduction in functional ability because of decreasing knee range of motion, making simple everyday tasks such as walking, climbing stairs, and getting in and out of a car quite difficult. (From Waldman SD. *Atlas of Common Pain Syndromes*. 4th ed. Philadelphia: Elsevier; 2019: Fig. 105.1.)

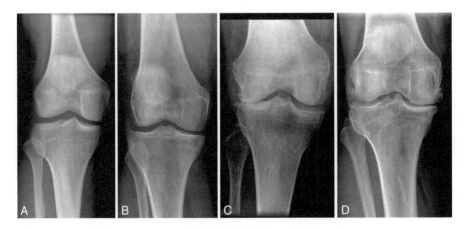

Fig. 1.6 X-rays of osteoarthritis of the knee: (A) grade 0 normal, (B) grade 1 lateral femoral osteophyte, (C) grade 2 lateral femoral osteophyte, and (D) grade 3 lateral femoral osteophyte. (From Altman RD, Gold GE. Atlas of individual radiographic features in osteoarthritis, revised. *Osteoarthr Cart*. 2007:15[1]:A1—A56 [Fig. 22].)

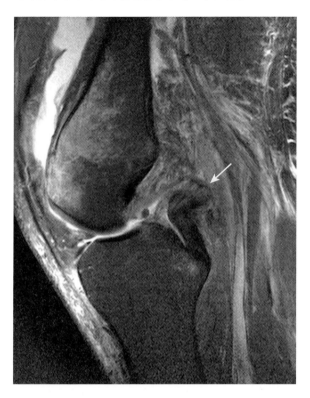

Fig. 1.7 Sagittal fat suppressed T2-weighted (FST2W) magnetic resonance (MR) image of an acute posterior cruciate ligament (PCL) tear. The proximal ligament is completely disrupted from its femoral attachment, and the torn end of the PCL is visualized *(white arrow)*. Note also the prominent trabecular bone bruising in the distal femur and the prominent joint effusion. (From Waldman SD, Campbell RSD. *Imaging of Pain*. Philadelphia: Saunders; 2011: Fig. 148.3.)

DIFFERENTIAL DIAGNOSIS

Many diseases can cause knee pain (Table 1.1). Lumbar radiculopathy may mimic the pain and disability associated with arthritis of the knee. In such patients, the knee examination should be negative. Bursitis of the knee and entrapment neuropathies such as meralgia paresthetica may also confuse the diagnosis; both these conditions may coexist with arthritis of the knee. Primary and metastatic tumors of the femur and spine may also present in a manner similar to arthritis of the knee.

TREATMENT

Initial treatment of the pain and functional disability associated with arthritis of the knee includes a combination of nonsteroidal antiinflammatory drugs or

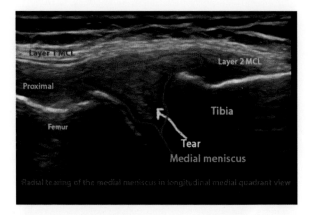

Fig. 1.8 Ultrasound image of the knee demonstrating a torn medial meniscus. (Courtesy Steven Waldman, MD.)

TABLE 1.1 ■ Causes of Knee Pain and Dysfunction

Arthritis
- Osteoarthritis
- Rheumatoid
- Gout
- Pseudogout
- Reactive arthritis
- Septic arthritis

Trauma
- Fractures
- Meniscal injuries
- Tendinitis
- Bursitis
- Ligamentous injuries

Mechanical Abnormalities
- Joint mouse
- Altered gait due to hip, foot, or ankle problems
- Iliotibial band syndrome
- Patellar abnormalities (e.g., patella alta, bipartite patella)

Other Causes
- Avascular necrosis
- Foreign-body synovitis
- Charcot joint
- Neurofibromatosis
- Malignancy
- Pseudorheumatism

cyclooxygenase-2 inhibitors and physical therapy. The local application of heat and cold may also be beneficial. For patients who do not respond to these treatment modalities, intraarticular injection of local anesthetic and steroid is a reasonable next step.

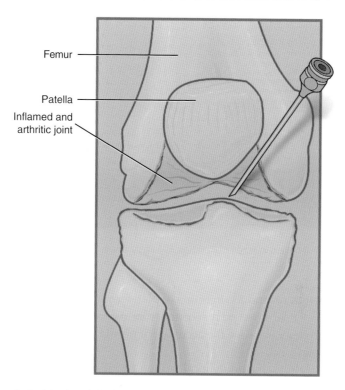

Femur

Patella

Inflamed and
arthritic joint

Fig 1.9 Intraarticular injection of the knee. (From Waldman SD. *Atlas of Pain Management Injection Techniques*. 4th ed. St Louis: Elsevier; 2017: Fig. 132-4.)

For intraarticular injection of the knee, the patient is placed in the supine position with a rolled blanket underneath the knee to gently flex the joint. The skin overlying the medial joint is prepared with antiseptic solution. A sterile syringe containing 5 mL of 0.25% preservative-free bupivacaine and 40 mg methylprednisolone is attached to a 1.5-inch, 25-gauge needle using strict aseptic technique. The joint space is identified, and the clinician places a thumb on the lateral margin of the patella and pushes it medially. At a point in the middle of the medial edge of the patella, the needle is inserted between the patella and the femoral condyles. The needle is then carefully advanced through the skin and subcutaneous tissues through the joint capsule and into the joint (Fig. 1.9). If bone is encountered, the needle is withdrawn into the subcutaneous tissues and redirected superiorly. After the joint space is entered, the contents of the syringe are gently injected. There should be little resistance to injection. If resistance is encountered, the needle is probably in a ligament or tendon and should be advanced slightly into the joint space until the injection can proceed without significant resistance. The needle is then removed, and a sterile pressure dressing and ice pack are applied to the injection site. Clinical studies suggest that

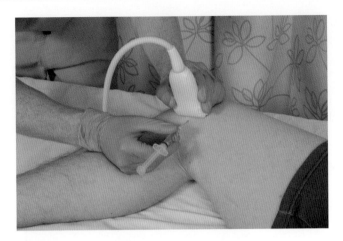

Fig. 1.10 Ultrasound-guided injection of the knee. (Courtesy Steven Waldman, MD.)

viscosupplementation and the injection of platelet-rich plasma may also provide symptomatic relief of knee pain secondary to osteoarthritis. The use of ultrasound guidance may improve the accuracy of needle placement into the intraarticular space (Fig. 1.10).

Physical modalities, including local heat and gentle range of motion exercises, should be introduced several days after the patient undergoes injection. Vigorous exercises should be avoided because they will exacerbate patient symptoms.

HIGH-YIELD TAKEAWAYS

- The patient is afebrile, making an acute infectious etiology (e.g., septic arthritis) unlikely.
- The patient's symptomatology is not the result of acute trauma but more likely the result of repetitive microtrauma that has damaged the joint over time.
- The patient's pain is diffuse rather than highly localized, as would be the case with a pathologic process such as prepatellar bursitis.
- The patient's symptoms are unilateral and involve only one joint, which is more suggestive of a local process than a systemic polyarthropathy.
- Sleep disturbance is common and must be addressed concurrently with the patient's pain symptomatology.
- Plain radiographs will provide high-yield information regarding the bony contents of the joint, but ultrasound imaging and MRI will be more useful in identifying soft tissue pathology.

Suggested Readings

Waldman SD. Arthritis and Other Abnormalities of the Knee. In: *Waldman's Comprehensive Atlas of Diagnostic Ultrasound of Painful Conditions*. Philadelphia: Wolters Kluwer; 2016:725–740.

Waldman SD. Functional Anatomy of the Knee. In: *Pain Review*. 2nd ed. Philadelphia: Elsevier; 2017:142–144.

Waldman SD. Intra-articular Injection of the Knee Joint. In: *Atlas of Pain Management Injection Techniques*. 4th ed. Philadelphia: Elsevier; 2017:487–490.

Waldman SD. Intra-articular injection of the knee joint. In: *Pain Review*. 2nd ed. Philadelphia: Elsevier; 2017:546–547.

Waldman SD, Campbell RSD. Anatomy, Special Imaging Considerations of the Knee. In: *Imaging of Pain*. Philadelphia: Saunders Elsevier; 2011:367–368.

Waldman SD, Campbell RSD. Osteonecrosis of the Knee. In: *Imaging of Pain*. Philadelphia: Saunders Elsevier; 2011:393–396.

Xu C, Peng H, Li R, et al. Risk factors and clinical characteristics of deep knee infection in patients with intra-articular injections: a matched retrospective cohort analysis. *Sem Arthr Rheum*. 2018;47(6):911–916.

Brendan Beckham

A 32-Year-Old Male With Acute Left Medial Knee Pain Following a Soccer Injury

LEARNING OBJECTIVES

- Learn the common causes of knee pain.
- Develop an understanding of the unique anatomy of the knee joint.
- Develop an understanding of the anatomy of the medial meniscus.
- Understand the function of the muscles of the medial meniscus.
- Develop an understanding of the causes of medial meniscus tear.
- Develop an understanding of the various types of medial meniscus injury.
- Learn the clinical presentation of medial meniscus tear.
- Learn how to examine the knee.
- Learn how to use physical examination to identify pathology of the medial meniscus.
- Develop an understanding of the treatment options for medial meniscus tear.

Brendan Beckham

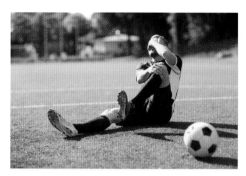

"Call me Brendan," my new patient said as I introduced myself. Brendan was a 28-year-old professional soccer player with our local farm team with the chief complaint of, "I blew out my right knee." Brendan stated that about a week ago, he was taking the ball down to the goal and pivoted to avoid a defender to move in for the score when he felt like "something popped in my left knee. Doc, it really hurt, but I went ahead and made the kick, scored, and then headed off to the locker room to ice my knee. I took a quick shower, but the inside of my knee was killing me. I didn't immediately say anything to anybody because, you know, at my age..." as his voiced just trailed off. "But I figured with ice, Tylenol, and a couple of days off, I would be right as rain. But here I am," he said with a weak smile. I asked if he had ever had anything like this before and he shook his head and said, "Just the usual aches and pains. I never miss a game. I love playing soccer. I hope to play for a long time yet, so I need you to give me a shot or something. No hard drugs, because the league is always doing drug screens."

I told Brendan I would do all I could for him, and the first step was to figure out exactly what was going on with his knee. I asked Brendan how he was sleeping and he said, "Pretty well, but every time I roll onto my left knee, I wake up." Brendan denied any fever or chills.

On physical examination, Brendan was afebrile. His respirations were 16 and his pulse was 64 and regular. His blood pressure was 118/82. His head, eyes, ears, nose, throat (HEENT) exam was normal, as was his cardiopulmonary examination. His thyroid was normal. His abdominal examination revealed no abnormal mass or organomegaly. There was a left lower quadrant scar that Brendan said was from an appendectomy when he was a kid. There was no costovertebral angle (CVA) tenderness. There was no peripheral edema. His low back examination was unremarkable. Visual inspection of the left knee revealed a small area of ecchymosis over the medial joint space. I asked Brendan about it and he said, "Oh, that's nothing, just a little bruising from the acupuncture." I asked if the acupuncture helped and he gave me a wry smile and said if it did, he would be at practice rather than sitting on my exam table.

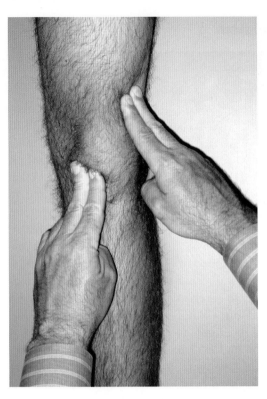

Fig. 2.1 Eliciting the bulge sign for small knee joint effusions. (From Waldman SD. *Physical Diagnosis of Pain: An Atlas of Signs and Symptoms*. 3rd ed. St Louis: Elsevier; 2016: Fig. 202-1.)

I asked Brendan to point with one finger to show me where it hurt the most, and he pointed to the area over the medial joint space. He said, "Doc, it feels like it's down in the knee; not on the outside." He volunteered, "Sometimes after a squat, when I get up, it feels like my knee is going to catch or lock up." I gently flexed and extended the knee and he said that reproduced the pain. The left knee was a little warm medially but did not appear to be infected. I felt like Brendan had a large joint effusion, so I performed the bulge sign test for knee joint effusions, which was positive, as was his ballottement test (Figs. 2.1–2.3). Brendan exhibited a positive McMurray test as well as a positive squat test (Figs. 2.4 and 2.5). Brendan's right knee examination was normal, as was examination of his other major joints. A careful neurologic examination of the upper and lower extremities revealed there was no evidence of peripheral or entrapment neuropathy, and the deep tendon reflexes were normal. I told Brendan I was pretty sure I knew what was going on and we were going to get some tests to confirm it.

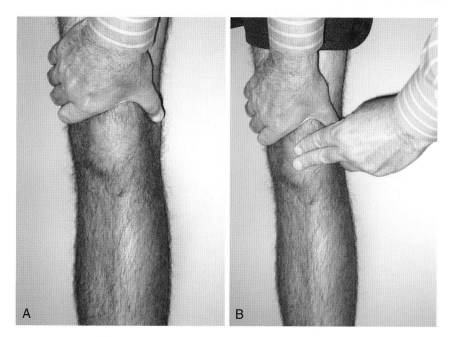

Fig. 2.2   Eliciting the ballottement sign for large knee joint effusions. (A) The examiner displaces synovial fluid from the suprapatellar pouch into the joint. (B) The examiner ballottes the patella. (From
Waldman SD. *Physical Diagnosis of Pain: An Atlas of Signs and Symptoms*. 3rd ed. St Louis: Elsevier;
2016: Fig. 203.1A,B.)

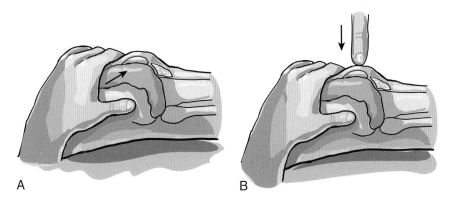

Fig. 2.3   The ballottement test. (A) The examiner displaces synovial fluid from the suprapatellar pouch
into the joint. (B) The examiner performs ballottement on the patella. (From Waldman SD. *Physical
Diagnosis of Pain: An Atlas of Signs and Symptoms*. 3rd ed. St Louis: Elsevier; 2016: Fig. 203.2A,B.)

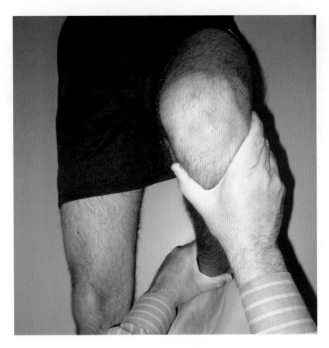

Fig. 2.4 The McMurray test for torn meniscus. (From Waldman SD. *Physical Diagnosis of Pain: An Atlas of Signs and Symptoms*. 3rd ed. St Louis: Elsevier; 2016: Fig. 219-1.)

Key Clinical Points—What's Important and What's Not

THE HISTORY

- A history of sudden onset left medial joint pain following a soccer injury
- A history of a sudden pop in the knee at the time of the acute injury
- A history of continued pain in spite of conservative therapy, including acupuncture
- No history of previous significant knee pain
- No fever or chills
- Sleep disturbance

THE PHYSICAL EXAMINATION

- The patient is afebrile
- Palpation of left knee reveals tenderness over the medial joint space
- An effusion of the left knee joint as indicated by a positive bulge and ballottement test

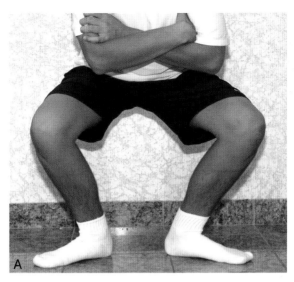

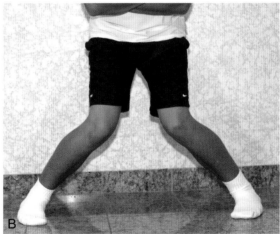

Fig. 2.5 The squat test for torn meniscus. (A) The squat test for meniscal tear. The patient is asked first to perform a full squat with the feet and legs fully externally rotated. (B) The squat test for meniscal tear. The patient is then asked to perform a full squat with the feet and legs fully internally rotated. (From Waldman SD. *Physical Diagnosis of Pain: An Atlas of Signs and Symptoms*. 3rd ed. St Louis: Elsevier; 2016 [Figs. 221-3 and 221-4].)

- The presence of mild ecchymosis over the medial right knee joint space
- Pain on flexion and extension of the left knee
- A positive drop McMurray test
- A positive squat test

OTHER FINDINGS OF NOTE

- Normal HEENT examination
- Normal cardiovascular examination
- Normal pulmonary examination
- Normal abdominal examination with a well-healed appendectomy scar noted
- No peripheral edema
- Normal upper extremity neurologic examination, motor and sensory examination
- Examination of other joints was normal

What Tests Would You Like to Order?

The following tests were ordered:
- Plain radiographs of the left knee
- Magnetic resonance imaging (MRI) of the left knee
- Ultrasound of the left knee with special attention to the medial meniscus

TEST RESULTS

The plain radiographs of the left knee revealed no evidence of bony abnormality or fracture, but showed patellar tilting due to the large effusion behind and around the patellar tendon (Fig. 2.6). The MRI revealed a bucket handle tear of the medial meniscus (Fig. 2.7). The ultrasound of the left medial meniscus reveals complex tearing of the meniscus (Fig. 2.8).

Clinical Correlation—Putting It All Together

What is the diagnosis?
- Bucket handle tear of the medial meniscus

The Science Behind the Diagnosis

ANATOMY OF THE MEDIAL MENISCUS

The medial meniscus is a crescent-shaped fibrocartilaginous band that spans the medial knee joint (Fig. 2.9). The function of the medial meniscus is to provide chondroprotection by reducing peak contact forces and friction between the femur and proximal tibia (Fig. 2.10). The medial mensicus is attached to the tibia by the coronary ligaments, which are also subject to traumatic injury (Fig. 2.11).

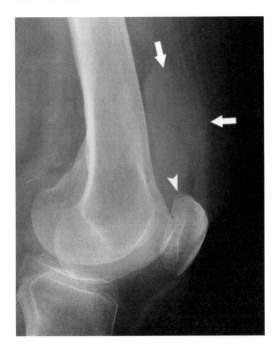

Fig. 2.6 Standing lateral radiograph demonstrating no evidence of bony abnormality, but with patellar tilting due to the large effusion behind and around the patellar tendon *(white arrows)*. (From Venkatasamy A, Ehlinger M, Bierry G. Acute traumatic knee radiographs: beware of lesions of little expression but of great significance. *Diagn Intervent Imaging.* 2014;95[6]:551–560 [fig. 3].)

CLINICAL CONSIDERATIONS

The meniscus is a unique anatomic structure that fulfills a variety of functions to allow ambulation in the upright position (Table 2.1). The meniscus is susceptible to both acute injury from trauma and degenerative tears, which are more chronic in nature. Tears of the medial meniscus are classified by their orientation and shape (Fig. 2.12; Table 2.2).

Acute medial meniscal injury is the most commonly encountered cause of significant knee pain secondary to trauma in clinical practice, with an incidence of acute tear of around 60 cases per 100,000 individuals. Acute tears often occur with sudden twisting or squatting with weight bearing (see Table 2.2). There is a male predominance of over 2:1. Medial meniscal tear is a disease of the third and forth decades in males and the second decade in females. In older patients, the incidence of degenerative medial meniscal tears approaches 60%, with not all of these tears causing significant pain and functional disability for the patient.

The pain of medial meniscal tear is characterized by pain at the medial aspect of the knee joint line. The medial meniscus is a triangular structure on cross

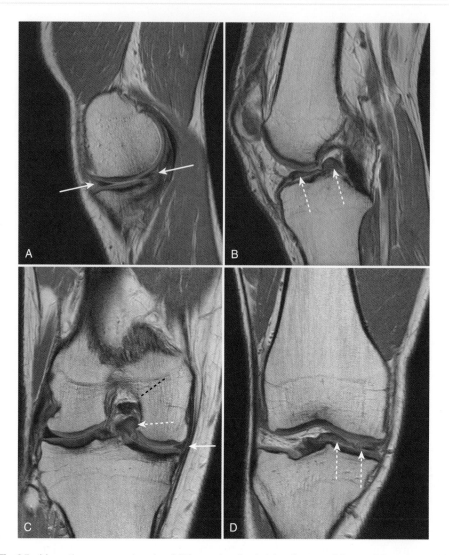

Fig. 2.7 Magnetic resonance imaging (MRI) reveals a bucket handle tear of the medial meniscus. (A) The parasagittal proton density MRI indicates a small meniscus *(white arrows)*. (B) The sagittal proton density MRI through the level of the intercondylar notch shows a displaced bucket handle fragment of the medial meniscus *(broken white arrows)* lying inferior and anterior to the posterior collateral ligament. (C) Full-thickness tear of the supraspinatus tendon as well as (D) more chronic tendinopathy of the infraspinatus tendon as evidenced by thickening and high signal intensity of the tendon. (From Waldman SD, Campbell RSD. *Imaging of Pain*. Philadelphia: Saunders; 2011: Fig. 146.2A,B.)

section, which is approximately 3.5 cm in length from anterior to posterior (see Fig. 2.10). It is wider posteriorly and is attached to the tibia by the coronary ligaments, which are also susceptible to trauma, as are the fibrous connections from the joint capsule and medial collateral ligament.

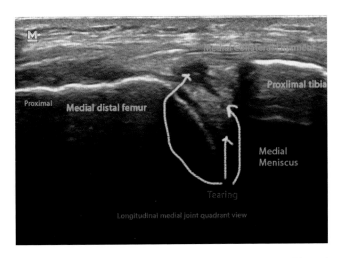

Fig. 2.8 Longitudinal ultrasound image revealing complex tearing of the medial meniscus. (Courtesy Steven Waldman, MD.)

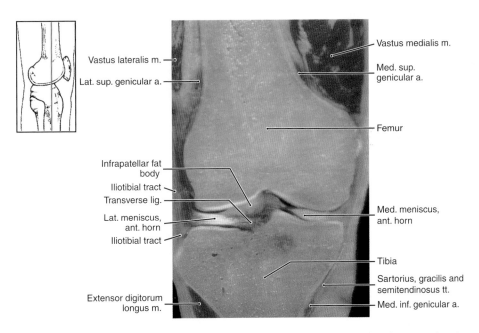

Fig. 2.9 The medial meniscus is subject to degenerative changes as well as tearing secondary to acute trauma. *m*, muscle; *a*, artery; *ant*, anterior; *tt*, tendons. (From Kang HS, Ahn JM, Resnick D. *MRI of the Extremities: An Anatomic Atlas*. 2nd ed. Philadelphia: Saunders; 2002:305.)

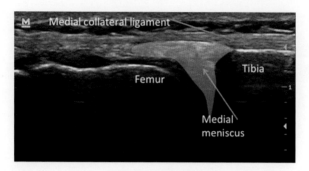

Fig. 2.10 Longitudinal ultrasound image demonstrating the triangular medial meniscus nestled between the medial borders of the femur and tibia. (Courtesy Steven Waldman, MD.)

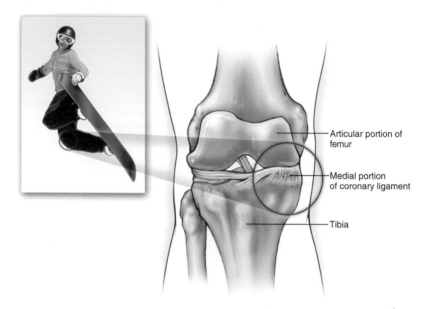

Fig. 2.11 The medial mensicus is attached to the tibia by the coronary ligaments, which are also subject to traumatic injury, which can result in medial knee pain. (From Waldman SD. *Atlas of Uncommon Pain Syndromes*. 3rd ed. Philadelphia: Saunders; 2014: Fig. 102-1.)

TABLE 2.1 ■ Functions of the Medial Meniscus

- Load bearing
- Converting the compressive forces to tensile forces
- Load distribution
- Stabilization of the joint
- Lubrication of the joint
- Proprioception

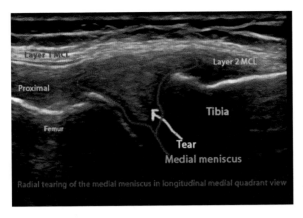

Fig. 2.12 Ultrasound image demonstrating a radial tear of the medial meniscus. (Courtesy Steven Waldman, MD.)

TABLE 2.2 ■ Classification of Tears of the Medial Meniscus

- Longitudinal tears
- Bucket handle tears
- Parrot beak–shaped oblique tears
- Horizontal tears
- Radial tears
- Complex combination tears

SIGNS AND SYMPTOMS

Patients with medial meniscal tear present with pain over the medial joint space and increased pain on the McMurray, squat, and Apley grinding tests (see Figs. 2.4 and 2.5). Activity, especially flexion and external rotation of the knee, makes the pain worse, whereas rest and heat provide some relief. The pain is constant and is characterized as aching in nature; it may interfere with sleep. Patients with injury to the medial meniscus may complain of locking or popping with flexion of the affected knee. An effusion is often present and can be quite pronounced in some patients. Coexistent bursitis, tendinitis, arthritis, or other internal derangement of the knee may confuse the clinical picture after trauma to the knee joint (Table 2.3).

On physical examination, patients with injury to the medial collateral ligament exhibit tenderness along the medial joint line. Patients with tear of the medial meniscus may exhibit positive McMurray, squat, and Apley tests. Because pain may produce muscle guarding, making accurate joint examination difficult, MRI of the knee may be necessary to confirm the clinical impression.

TABLE 2.3 ■ Most Common Causes of Knee Pain

Localized Bony or Joint Space Pathology	Periarticular Pathology	Systemic Disease	Sympathetically Mediated Pain	Referred From Other Body Areas
Fracture	Bursitis	Rheumatoid	Causalgia	Lumbar
Primary bone tumor	Tendinitis	arthritis	Reflex sympathetic	plexopathy
Primary synovial tis-	Adhesive capsulitis	Collagen vascular	dystrophy	Lumbar
sue tumor	Joint instability	disease		radiculopathy
Joint instability	Muscle strain	Reiter syndrome		Lumbar
Localized arthritis	Muscle sprain	Gout		spondylosis
Osteophyte	Periarticular infection	Other crystal		Fibromyalgia
formation	not involving	arthropathies		Myofascial pain
Joint space infection	joint space	Charcot neuro-		syndromes
Hemarthrosis		pathic arthritis		Inguinal hernia
Villonodular synovitis				Entrapment
Intraarticular foreign				neuropathies
body				Intrapelvic tumors
Osgood-Schlatter				Retroperitoneal
disease				tumors
Chronic dislocation				
of the patella				
Patellofemoral pain				
syndrome				
Patella alta				

From Waldman SD. *Physical Diagnosis of Pain: An Atlas of Signs and Symptoms*. 3rd ed. St Louis: Elsevier; 2016: Table 201-1.

TESTING

Plain radiographs and MRI are indicated in all patients who present with knee pain, particularly if internal derangement or occult mass or tumor is suspected (Fig. 2.13). In addition, MRI should be performed in all patients with injury to the medial meniscus who fail to respond to conservative therapy or who exhibit joint instability on clinical examination. Bone scan may be useful to identify occult stress fractures involving the joint, especially if trauma has occurred. Based on the patient's clinical presentation, additional testing may be warranted, including a complete blood count, erythrocyte sedimentation rate, and antinuclear antibody testing.

DIFFERENTIAL DIAGNOSIS

Any condition affecting the medial compartment of the knee joint may mimic the pain of medial meniscal tear. Bursitis, arthritis, and entrapment neuropathies may also confuse the diagnosis, as may primary tumors of the knee and spine.

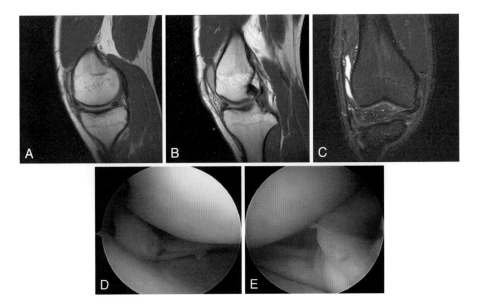

Fig. 2.13 (A–C) Sagittal proton density magnetic resonance imaging (MRI) demonstrating a horizontal tear of the medial meniscal body with an anterior horn fragment displaced anterior to the medial femoral condyle (A) and a posterior horn fragment displaced into the intercondylar notch adjacent to the posterior cruciate ligament (B). Both displaced fragments were missed on MRI. (C) Coronal short tau inversion recovery (STIR) MRI also demonstrating the displaced anterior horn meniscal fragment mentioned in (A). This fragment was palpable to the patient, who brought it to the attention of the surgeon before arthroscopy. (D, E) Arthroscopic images of the same case demonstrating the horizontal tear of the meniscal body and the displaced posterior horn (D) and anterior horn fragments (E). (From Sampson MJ, Jackson MP, Moran CJ, et al. Three tesla MRI for the diagnosis of meniscal and anterior cruciate ligament pathology: a comparison to arthroscopic findings. *Clin Radiol.* 2008;63 [10]:1106–1111.)

TREATMENT

Initial treatment of the pain and functional disability associated with injury to the medial collateral ligament includes a combination of nonsteroidal antiinflammatory drugs or cyclooxygenase-2 inhibitors and physical therapy. The local application of heat and cold may also be beneficial. Any repetitive activity that exacerbates the patient's symptoms should be avoided. For patients who do not respond to these treatment modalities and do not have lesions that require surgical repair, injection with local anesthetic and steroid is a reasonable next step. Ultrasound guidance will increase the accuracy of needle placement (Fig. 2.14).

Physical modalities, including local heat and gentle range of motion exercises, should be introduced several days after the patient undergoes injection. Vigorous exercises should be avoided because they will exacerbate patient symptoms.

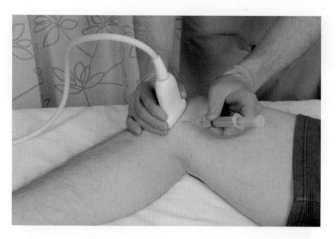

Fig. 2.14   Ultrasound-guided medial meniscus injection. (Courtesy Steven Waldman, MD.)

HIGH-YIELD TAKEAWAYS

- The patient is afebrile, making an acute infectious etiology (e.g., septic arthritis) unlikely.
- The patient's symptomatology is the result of a soccer injury, and testing should be focused on the identification of ligamentous injury and fracture.
- The patient's pain is localized to the medial joint space.
- The patient's symptoms are unilateral and involve only one joint, which is more suggestive of a local process than a systemic polyarthropathy.
- Sleep disturbance is common and must be addressed concurrently with the patient's pain symptomatology.
- Plain radiographs will provide high-yield information regarding the bony contents of the joint, but ultrasound imaging and MRI will be more useful in identifying soft tissue pathology.

Suggested Readings

Allen H, Chan BY, Davis KW, et al. Overuse injuries of the knee. *Radiol Clin North Am.* 2019;58(5):898—909.

Cibulas A, Leyva A, Cibulas G, et al. Acute knee injury. *Radiol Clin North Am.* 2019;58 (5):883—898.

Netter FH. Knee (glenohumeral joint). In: *Atlas of Human Anatomy.* 4th ed. Philadelphia: Saunders; 2008.

Waldman SD. Atlas of Pain Management Injection Techniques. 4th ed. Philadelphia: Saunders; 2018:94—98.

Waldman SD. Clinical Correlates: Diseases of the Medial Meniscus. In: *Physical Diagnosis of Pain: An Atlas of Signs and Symptoms*. 3rd ed. Philadelphia: Elsevier; 2016:87–92.

Waldman SD. Clinical Correlates: Functional Anatomy of the knee. In: *Physical Diagnosis of Pain: An Atlas of Signs and Symptoms*. 3rd ed. Philadelphia: Saunders; 2018.

Waldman SD. Medial Meniscus Disease. In: *Waldman's Comprehensive Atlas of Diagnostic Ultrasound of Painful Conditions*. Philadelphia: Wolters Kluwer; 2016:186–195.

Waldman SD. Medial Meniscus Tear. In: *Atlas of Common Pain Syndromes*. 4th ed. Philadelphia: Elsevier; 2019:129–133.

Tony Garcia

A 24-Year-Old Male Football Player With Severe Posterior Knee Pain

- Learn the common causes of knee pain.
- Learn the common causes of semimembranosus insertion syndrome.
- Develop an understanding of the anatomy of the semimembranosus muscle.
- Develop an understanding of the differential diagnosis of semimembranosus insertion syndrome.
- Learn the clinical presentation of semimembranosus insertion syndrome.
- Learn how to examine the knee.
- Learn how to examine the semimembranosus muscle.
- Learn how to use physical examination to identify semimembranosus insertion syndrome.
- Develop an understanding of the treatment options for semimembranosus insertion syndrome.

Tony Garcia

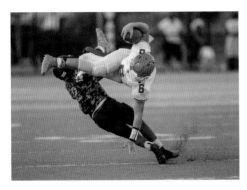

Tony Garcia is a 24-year-old football player with the chief complaint of, "I can't play because my knee is killing me." Tony stated that his problems begin during last Sunday's game when "that hoople head cut blocked me. The bad part was that jackass didn't even get a penalty! I limp off the field while he stands there laughing. Doc, it's been almost a week and my knee just isn't getting any better, even though I've been living in the whirlpool. The Advil, topical analgesic balm, and ice packs aren't touching it, either." He stated that usually when he gets injured, he just tries to "burn through it" because he doesn't want to "mess with my routine." Tony noted that the pain was made worse with weight bearing and walking. "Doc, I can barely get in and out of my SUV because of the pain." I asked Tony how he was sleeping and he shook his head and said, "Not worth a crap. I'm really getting worn out." I asked Tony if he ever had anything like this happen in the past and he said, "Not really, just the usual postgame aches and pains. It goes with the territory. We spend all the time between games just trying to heal for the next game. It's just part of the deal—muscle strains that go along with staying fit." I asked if he was experiencing any numbness or weakness and he shook his head no. "But you know, Doc, there is this one spot that hurts about as bad as a spot can hurt. It's really weirding me out." I said, "Show me the spot," and Tony pointed to a spot in the posterior medial knee and said, "Right here, Doc. If I hadn't had an X-ray, I would be sure that I fractured it." I reassured him that we would get things figured out, and then I asked Tony about any fever, chills, or other constitutional symptoms such as weight loss, night sweats, etc., and he just shook his head no.

On physical examination, Tony was afebrile. His respirations were 16, his pulse was 66 and regular, and his blood pressure was 112/68. Tony's head, eyes, ears, nose, throat (HEENT) exam was normal, as was his cardiopulmonary examination. His thyroid was normal. He was well muscled. His abdominal examination revealed no abnormal mass or organomegaly. There was no costovertebral angle (CVA) tenderness. There was no peripheral edema. His low back examination was unremarkable. Visual inspection of the right knee revealed resolving ecchymosis. There was no rubor, obvious infection, or bursitis. Palpation of the medial aspect posterior knee revealed

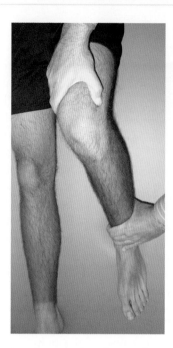

Fig. 3.1 The twist test for semimembranosus insertion syndrome. (From Waldman SD. *Physical Diagnosis of Pain: An Atlas of Signs and Symptoms*. 4th ed. Philadelphia: Elsevier; 2021: Fig 253.2.)

point tenderness over the distal insertion of the semimembranosus muscle on the medial surface of the medial condyle of the tibia. Tony exhibited a positive semimembranosus twist test (Fig. 3.1).

The left knee examination was normal. A careful neurologic examination of the upper extremities was completely normal. Deep tendon reflexes were normal.

Key Clinical Points—What's Important and What's Not

THE HISTORY

- A history of onset of right posterior knee pain following being tackled while playing football
- No numbness
- No weakness
- No history of previous significant knee pain
- No fever or chills
- Sleep disturbance

- Pain on getting in and out of car
- Pain on weightbearing and walking

THE PHYSICAL EXAMINATION

- The patient is afebrile
- Point tenderness over the insertion of the semimembranosus muscle on the medial tibial condyle
- Positive semimembranosus twist test
- Resolving ecchymosis over the posterior knee
- No obvious bursitis
- No obvious infection

OTHER FINDINGS OF NOTE

- Normal HEENT examination
- Normal cardiovascular examination
- Normal pulmonary examination
- Normal abdominal examination
- No peripheral edema
- Normal upper extremity neurologic examination, motor and sensory examination

 What Tests Would You Like to Order?

The following tests were ordered:
- Plain radiographs of the right knee
- Ultrasound of the right knee
- Magnetic resonance imaging (MRI) of the right knee

TEST RESULTS

The plain radiographs of the right knee revealed no evidence of bony abnormality or fracture. Ultrasound examination of the right knee revealed partial tearing of the semimembranosus tendon (Fig. 3.2). MRI scan of the right knee reveals edema of the tibial insertions of the semimembranosus muscle (Fig. 3.3).

 Clinical Correlation—Putting It All Together

What is the diagnosis?
- Semimembranosus insertion syndrome

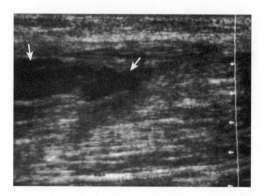

Fig. 3.2 Longitudinal ultrasound image demonstrating anechoic hemorrhage within the semimembranosus tendon. (From Waldman SD. *Atlas of Pain Management Injection Techniques*. 4th ed. St Louis: Elsevier; 2017: Fig. 135-7A.)

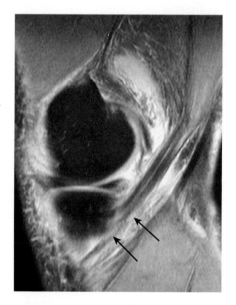

Fig. 3.3 Magnetic resonance imaging scan of the right knee reveals edema of the tibial insertions of semimembranosus muscle (*black arrows*). (From Waldman SD. *Atlas of Uncommon Pain Syndromes*. 3rd ed. Philadelphia: Saunders; 2014: Fig. 101-4C.)

The Science Behind the Diagnosis

ANATOMY

The semimembranosus muscle has its origin from the ischial tuberosity and inserts into a groove on the medial surface of the medial condyle of the tibia (Figs. 3.4 and 3.5). The semimembranosus muscle flexes and medially rotates

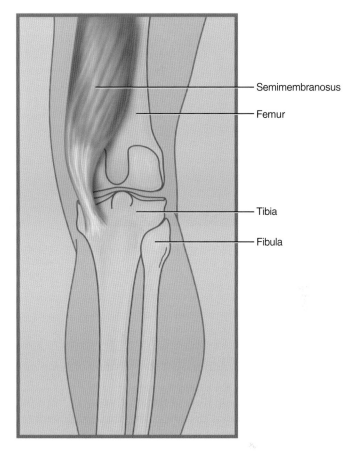

Fig. 3.4 The semimembranosus muscle has its origin from the ischial tuberosity and inserts into a groove on the medial surface of the medial condyle of the tibia. (From Waldman SD. *Atlas of Pain Management Injection Techniques*. 4th ed. St Louis: Elsevier; 2017: Fig. 135-2.)

the leg at the knee and extends the thigh at the hip joint. A fibrous extension of the muscle called the oblique popliteal ligament extends upward and laterally to provide support to the posterior knee joint. This ligament and the tendinous insertion of the muscle are prone to development of inflammation from overuse, misuse, or trauma. The semimembranosus muscle is innervated by the tibial portion of the sciatic nerve. The common peroneal nerve is in proximity to the insertion of the semimembranosus muscle, with the tibial nerve lying more medial. The popliteal artery and vein also lie in the middle of the joint. Also serving as a source of pain in the posterior knee is the semimembranosus bursa, which lies between the medial head of the gastrocnemius muscle, the medial femoral epicondyle, and the semimembranosus tendon (Fig. 3.6).

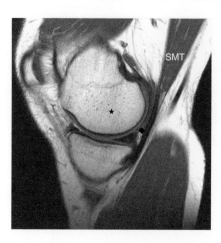

Fig. 3.5 Magnetic resonance imaging of the right knee *(sagittal)*: relationship between the semimembranosus tendon (SMT) and the medial femoral condyle *(star)*. (From von Dercks N, Theopold JD, Marquass B, et al. Snapping knee syndrome caused by semitendinosus and semimembranosus tendons. A case report. *Knee.* 2016;23[6]:1168–1171 [Fig. 2].)

CLINICAL SYNDROME

Semimembranosus insertion syndrome is a constellation of symptoms, including a localized tenderness over the posterior aspect of the medial knee joint with severe pain being elicited on palpation of the attachment of the semimembranosus muscle at the posterior medial condyle of the tibia. Semimembranosus insertion syndrome occurs most commonly after overuse or misuse of the knee, often after overaggressive exercise regimens. Direct trauma to the posterior knee by kicks or tackles during football also may result in the development of semimembranosus insertion syndrome (Fig. 3.7). Coexistent inflammation of the semimembranosus bursa that lies between the medial head of the gastrocnemius muscle, the medial femoral epicondyle, and the semimembranosus tendon may exacerbate the pain of semimembranosus insertion syndrome.

SIGNS AND SYMPTOMS

On physical examination, the patient exhibits point tenderness over the attachment of the semimembranosus muscle at the posterior medial condyle of the tibia. The patient may feel tenderness over the posterior knee and exhibits a positive twist test for semimembranosus insertion syndrome (see Fig. 3.1). The twist test is performed by placing the knee in 20 degrees of flexion and passively rotating the flexed knee. The test is positive if the pain is reproduced. Internal derangement of the knee also may be present and should be searched for on examination of the knee.

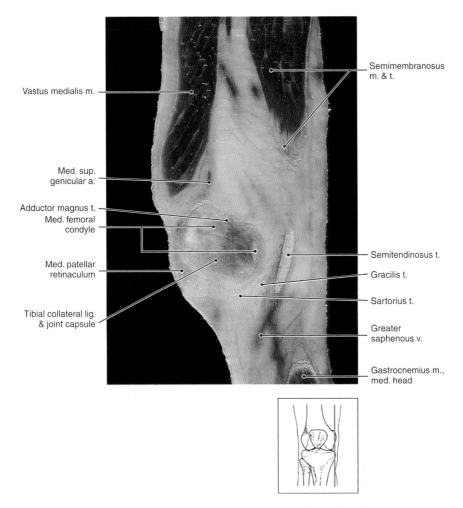

Fig. 3.6 Anatomy of the semimembranosus muscle tendon. a., Artery; *lig.*, ligament; *m.*, muscle; *med.*, medial; *sup.*, superior; *t.*, tendon; *v.*, vein. (From Kang HS, Ahn JM, Resnick D. *MRI of the Extremities: An Anatomic Atlas.* 2nd ed. Philadelphia: Saunders; 2002.)

TESTING

Plain radiographs are indicated in all patients who present with pain thought to be emanating from semimembranosus insertion syndrome to rule out occult bony pathology, including tibial plateau fractures and tumor (Fig. 3.8). Based on the patient's clinical presentation, additional tests may be indicated, including complete blood count, prostate-specific antigen, sedimentation rate, and antinuclear antibody testing. MRI, computed tomography, and ultrasound imaging of the knee are indicated if internal

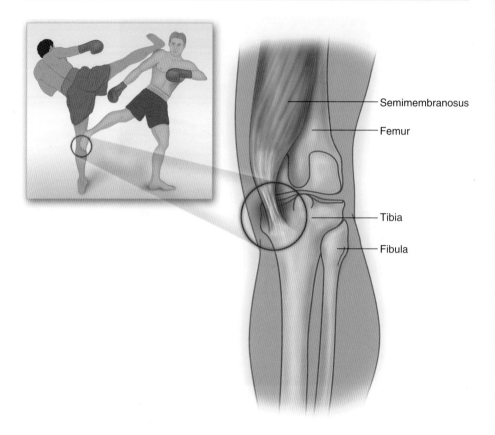

Fig. 3.7 Direct trauma to the posterior knee by kicks or tackles may cause semimembranosus insertion syndrome to develop. Semimembranosus insertion syndrome is a constellation of symptoms, including localized tenderness over the posterior aspect of the medial knee joint, with severe pain elicited on palpation of the attachment of the semimembranosus muscle at the posterior medial condyle of the tibia. (Modified from Waldman SD. *Atlas of Pain Management Injection Techniques*. 3rd ed. Philadelphia: Saunders; 2013:353.)

derangement, occult mass, or tumor is suspected as well as to confirm the diagnosis of semimembranosus insertion syndrome (Figs. 3.9 and 3.10). Radionucleotide bone scanning may be useful to rule out stress fractures not seen on plain radiographs. Injection of the semimembranosus insertions with local anesthetic and steroid may serve as both a diagnostic and a therapeutic maneuver.

DIFFERENTIAL DIAGNOSIS

Internal derangement of the knee and a ruptured Baker cyst may mimic the clinical presentation of semimembranosus insertion syndrome

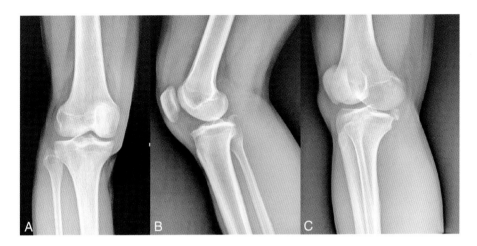

Fig. 3.8 A 23-year-old male patient reported a knee injury while he was playing soccer. (A) Anteroposterior X-ray view showing an anterolateral depression fracture. (B) Lateral X-ray view with a posteromedial tibial plateau fracture. (C) A 30-degree extrarotated lateral view with a better visualization of the fragment. (From Caggiari G, Ciurlia E, Ortu S, et al. Osteochondral avulsion fracture of the posteromedial tibial plateau. *Trauma Case Rep*. 2020;25:100281 [Fig. 1].)

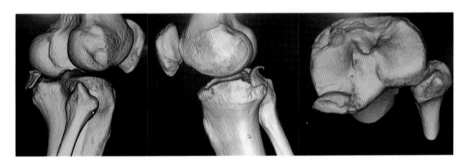

Fig. 3.9 Computed tomography images delineating the displaced fragment. Note that the displaced fragment has rotated 90 degrees in the sagittal plane. (From Caggiari G, Ciurlia E, Ortu S, et al. Osteochondral avulsion fracture of the posteromedial tibial plateau. *Trauma Case Rep*. 2020;25:100281 [Fig. 3].)

(Fig. 3.11). If trauma has occurred, the possibility of occult tibial plateau fracture, especially in patients with osteopenia or osteoporosis, should be considered, and radionucleotide bone scanning should be obtained. Villonodular synovitis and hemarthrosis of the knee may produce knee pain that can mimic the clinical presentation of semimembranosus insertion syndrome. Entrapment neuropathy or stretch injury, or both, to the

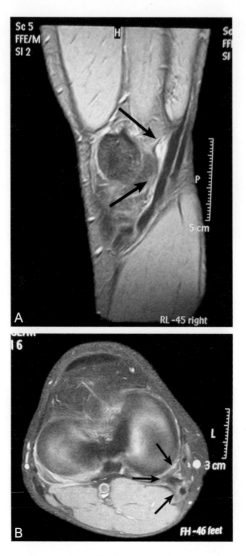

Fig. 3.10 (a) Magnetic resonance imaging (MRI) *(sagittal view)* showing existence of fluid in the semi-membranosus bursa and the sheath surrounding the semitendinosus and gracilis *(arrows)* (Philips Intera 1.5 T, Philips Medical Systems Holland BV, Sequence: T2 WFFE). (b) MRI *(transverse view)* showing fluid in the semimembranosus bursa and surrounding oedematous fat *(arrows)*. (From Karataglis D, Papadopoulos P, Fotiadou A, et al. Snapping knee syndrome in an athlete caused by the semitendinosus and gracilis tendons. A case report. *Knee.* 2008;15[2]:151—154 [Fig. 1].)

tibial branch of the sciatic nerve and common peroneal nerve, plexopathy, and radiculopathy should be considered if there is the physical finding of neurologic deficit in patients thought to have semimembranosus insertion syndrome, because all of these clinical entities may coexist.

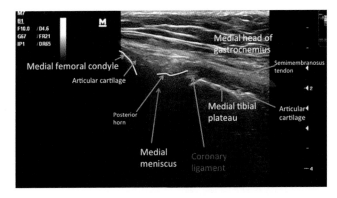

Fig. 3.11 Longitudinal ultrasound image demonstrating the relationship of the medial meniscus, coronary ligaments, and semimembranosus tendon. (Courtesy Steven Waldman, MD.)

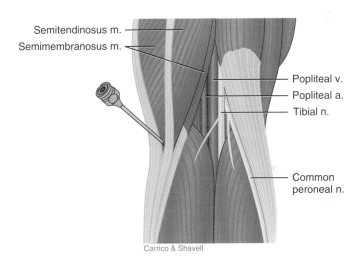

Fig. 3.12 Injection technique for semimembranosus insertion syndrome. (From Waldman SD. *Atlas of Pain Management Injection Techniques*. 4th ed. St Louis: Elsevier; 2017: Fig. 135-5.)

TREATMENT

Initial treatment of the pain and functional disability associated with semi-membranosus insertion syndrome should include a combination of nonsteroidal antiinflammatory drugs or cyclooxygenase-2 inhibitors and physical therapy. Local application of heat and cold may be beneficial. For patients who do not respond to these treatment modalities, injection of the semimembranosus insertion with a local anesthetic and steroid may be a reasonable next step (Fig. 3.12).

HIGH-YIELD TAKEAWAYS

- The patient is afebrile, making an acute infectious etiology unlikely.
- The patient's symptomatology is thought to be the result of overuse injury to the right semimembranosus muscle.
- Physical examination and testing should be focused on the identification of the various causes of semimembranosus insertion syndrome.
- The patient exhibits physical examination findings that are highly suggestive of semimembranosus insertion syndrome.
- The patient's symptoms are unilateral, suggestive of a local process rather than a systemic inflammatory process.
- Plain radiographs will provide high-yield information regarding the bony contents of the joint, but ultrasound imaging and MRI will be more useful in identifying soft tissue pathology that may be responsible for semimembranosus muscle compromise.

Suggested Readings

Waldman SD. Anatomy, Special Imaging Considerations of the Semimembranosus Insertion. In: *Imaging of Pain*. Philadelphia, PA: Elsevier; 2011:367–368.

Waldman SD. Functional Anatomy of the Semimembranosus Insertion. In: *Pain Review*. Philadelphia, PA: Saunders; 2009:144–149.

Waldman SD. Intra-articular Injection of the Semimembranosus Insertion Joint. In: *Atlas of Pain Management Injection Techniques*. ed 3 Philadelphia, PA: Elsevier; 2013:346–348.

Waldman SD. Intra-articular Injection of the Semimembranosus Insertion Joint. In: *Pain Review*. Philadelphia, PA: Saunders; 2009:583–584.

Waldman SD. Ultrasound-guided Injection Technique for Semimembranosus Insertion Syndrome. In: *Comprehensive Atlas of Ultrasound Guided Pain Management Injection Techniques*. ed 2 Philadelphia, PA: Wolters Kluwer; 2020:721–725.

Waldman SD, Campbell RSD. Osteonecrosis of the Semimembranosus Insertion. In: *Imaging of Pain*. Philadelphia, PA: Elsevier; 2011:393–396.

Miller Maier

A 24-Year-Old Male With a Painful, Unsteady Right Knee Following a Skiing Accident

LEARNING OBJECTIVES

- Learn the common causes of knee pain.
- Develop an understanding of the unique anatomy of the knee joint.
- Develop an understanding of the bursae of the knee.
- Develop an understanding of the ligaments of the knee.
- Develop an understanding of the tendons of the knee.
- Develop an understanding of the differential diagnosis of knee pain.
- Learn the clinical presentation of anterior cruciate ligament injury.
- Learn how to examine the knee and associated ligaments.
- Learn how to use physical examination to identify anterior cruciate ligament injury.
- Develop an understanding of the treatment options for anterior cruciate ligament injury.

Miller Maier

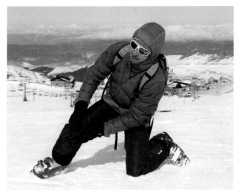

Miller Maier is a 24-year-old accountant with the chief complaint of, "My right knee keeps giving out." Miller stated that he was snow skiing at Big Bear last weekend when his right ski tip dug in, twisting his knee and causing him to fall "halfway down the mountain." He said he heard a loud pop from his right knee as soon as his ski tip dug in. Miller said he was pretty shook up, so he just lay there for a while. When he got up, his right knee really hurt, but what really scared him was that he had a feeling that the knee was slipping backward. Miller said that by the time he got home, he had a huge bruise on the front of his right knee and it was swollen up about twice its normal size. He elevated his leg and used an ice pack, which seemed to help the swelling, but the "slipping backward" sensation and the knee pain continued. He took some of his partner's pain pills, but all they did was make him feel like he was going to throw up all the time.

"Doctor, this crazy, unsteady feeling in my knee is really driving me crazy. At first I thought I just sprained it, and it would get better, but if anything the 'slipping backward' feeling is getting worse." I asked Miller about any previous injuries to the right knee and he said, "In fact, I'm a damn good skier and have never had a serious fall. Doc, I can tough it through the pain, but the unsteady knee is really freaking me out. What the hell did I do to my knee?"

I asked Miller what made his symptoms worse and he said, "Anytime I put any weight on my right knee, I'm in trouble. I have been walking so funny that now my left knee is starting to bother me. Doctor, my knee is hurting all the time and the pain is really messing with my sleep because I just can't seem to find a comfortable position. Every time I roll over onto my right side, the pain in my knee wakes me up."

I asked Miller to point with one finger to show me where the snap came from and he pointed to the area in front of his right knee, just below the patella, and said, "Right here, Doc."

On physical examination, Miller was afebrile. His respirations were 18 and his pulse was 64 and regular. His blood pressure was 118/40. His head, eyes, ears, nose, and throat (HEENT) exam was normal, as was his cardiopulmonary examination. His thyroid was normal, as was his abdominal examination. There was no costovertebral angle (CVA) tenderness. There was no peripheral edema. His low back examination was unremarkable. Visual inspection of the right knee

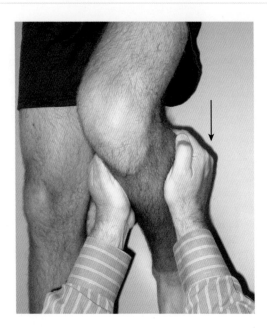

Fig. 4.1 The anterior drawer test for anterior cruciate integrity. (From Waldman SD. *Physical Diagnosis of Pain: An Atlas of Signs and Symptoms*. 3rd ed. St Louis: Elsevier; 2016: Fig. 206-1].)

revealed a resolving ecchymosis and moderate swelling. The area over the anterior knee was warm but did not appear to be infected. There was some tenderness with palpation of the patellar tendon. Examination of the bursae of the knee revealed no obvious bursitis. I performed an anterior drawer test, which was markedly positive on the right and negative on the left (Fig. 4.1). The Lachman test for anterior cruciate ligament integrity was also positive (Fig. 4.2). Range of motion of the knee joint, especially resisted extension of the joint, reproduced Miller's pain. The left knee examination was normal as was examination of his other major joints. A careful neurologic examination of the upper and lower extremities revealed that there was no evidence of peripheral or entrapment neuropathy, and the deep tendon reflexes were normal.

Key Clinical Points—What's Important and What's Not
THE HISTORY

- Onset of right knee pain and a backward sliding sensation of the knee following a ski injury
- An audible popping sound from the right knee at the time of injury

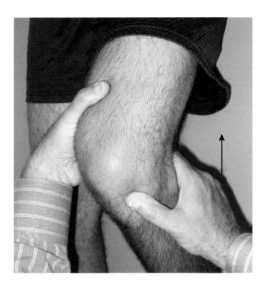

Fig. 4.2 The Lachman test for anterior cruciate integrity. (From Waldman SD. *Physical Diagnosis of Pain: An Atlas of Signs and Symptoms*. 3rd ed. St Louis, MO: Elsevier; 2016: Fig 208-1.)

- Pain localized to the anterior knee
- No other specific traumatic event to the area identified
- No fever or chills
- Sleep disturbance

THE PHYSICAL EXAMINATION

- The patient is afebrile
- There is a resolving ecchymosis over the anterior knee
- There is moderate swelling of the knee
- Tenderness to palpation of the patellar tendon on the right
- No evidence of infection
- Pain on resisted extension of the affected right knee
- The anterior drawer test was positive on the right (see Fig. 4.1)
- The Lachman test was positive on the right (see Fig. 4.2)

OTHER FINDINGS OF NOTE

- Normal HEENT examination
- Normal cardiovascular examination
- Normal pulmonary examination

- Normal abdominal examination
- No peripheral edema
- Normal upper and lower extremity neurologic examination, motor and sensory examination
- No evidence of bursitis
- Examinations of joints other than the right knee were normal

What Tests Would You Like to Order?

The following tests were ordered:
- Plain radiographs of the right knee
- Ultrasound of the right knee
- Magnetic resonance imaging (MRI) of the right knee

TEST RESULTS

The plain radiographs of the right knee were reported as normal. Ultrasound examination of the right knee revealed complete disruption of the anterior cruciate ligament (Fig. 4.3). MRI examination of the right knee demonstrated complete disruption of the anterior cruciate ligament with retraction from the femoral attachment site (Fig. 4.4).

Clinical Correlation—Putting It All Together

What is the diagnosis?
- Ruptured anterior cruciate ligament

The Science Behind the Diagnosis

ANATOMY

The anterior cruciate ligament controls the amount of anterior movement or translation of the tibia relative to the femur and provides important proprioceptive information regarding the position of the knee. It is made up of dense fibroelastic fibers that run from the posteriomedial surface of the lateral condyle of the distal femur via the intercondylar notch to the anterior surface of the tibia (Figs. 4.5 and 4.6). The anterior cruciate ligament is innervated by the posterior branch of the posterior tibial nerve. The ligament is susceptible to sprain or partial or complete tear.

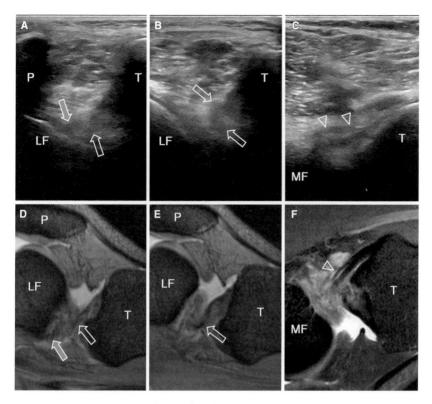

Fig. 4.3 Ultrasound examinations and magnetic resonance imaging of the traumatic knee of the patient. Long-axis view of the anterior cruciate ligament (ACL) (A, B) and posterior cruciate ligament (PCL) (C). Complete disruption at the proximal ACL with retraction with discontinuity between femoral attachment site (*arrow*, B) of the ACL and distal torn fragments (*open arrows*, A and B) is observed, indicating complete ACL rupture. In addition, partial disruption (*arrowheads*, C) of the continuity at the mid-PCL without retraction is observed, indicating partial PCL rupture. (D, E) Sagittal T1 multiple fast-field echo images show complete disruption at the proximal ACL with retraction with discontinuity between femoral attachment site (*arrow*, E) of the ACL and distal torn fragments (*open arrows*, D and E). (F) Sagittal proton density fat-suppressed image shows partial disruption *(arrowhead)* of the mid-PCL. These lesions correlated well with findings of point-of-care ultrasound examinations. *LF*, Lateral femoral condyle; *MF*, medial femoral condyle; *P*, patella; *T*, tibia. (From Lee SH, Yun SJ. Diagnosis of simultaneous acute ruptures of the anterior cruciate ligament and posterior cruciate ligament using point-of-care ultrasound in the emergency department. *J Emerg Med.* 2018;54(3):335–338 [Fig 2].)

CLINICAL SYNDROME

Anterior cruciate ligament syndrome is characterized by pain in the anterior aspect of the knee joint. It is usually the result of trauma to the anterior cruciate ligament from sudden deceleration due to the planting of the affected lower

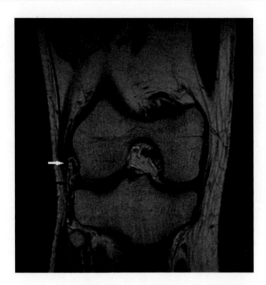

Fig. 4.4 Proton density-weighted coronal image of a 30-year-old male with anterior cruciate ligament (ACL) rupture. The femoral *(white arrow)* and tibial *(black arrow)* portions are visualized in image. The meniscal portion is not visualized in coronal image. (From Duran S, Gunaydin E, Aksahin E, et al. Evaluation of the anterolateral ligament of the knee by magnetic resonance imaging in patients with chronic anterior cruciate ligament rupture. *J Clin Orthop Trauma.* 2019;10(4):706–709, Fig. 2.)

extremity while extreme twisting or hyperextension forces are placed on the knee, typically during snow skiing accidents and football or basketball injuries (Fig. 4.7). Unlike many other painful knee syndromes, anterior cruciate ligament syndrome occurs significantly more frequently in females.

SIGNS AND SYMPTOMS

Patients with anterior cruciate ligament syndrome present with pain over the anterior knee joint and increased pain on passive valgus stress and range of motion of the knee. Activity makes the pain worse, whereas rest and heat provide some relief. The pain is constant and is characterized as aching in nature; it may interfere with sleep. Patients with injury to the anterior cruciate ligament may complain of a sudden popping of the affected knee at the time of acute injury as well as a sensation that the knee wants to give way or slip backwards. Coexistent bursitis, tendinitis, arthritis, or internal derangement of the knee may confuse the clinical picture after trauma to the knee joint. It should be noted that there is often injury to the menisci of the knee when the patient sustains knee trauma severe enough to disrupt the anterior cruciate ligament.

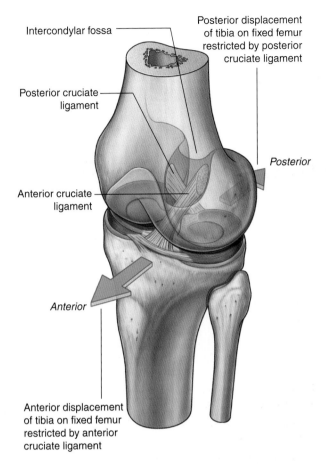

Intercondylar fossa

Posterior displacement
of tibia on fixed femur
restricted by posterior
cruciate ligament

Posterior cruciate
ligament

Posterior

Anterior cruciate
ligament

Anterior

Anterior displacement
of tibia on fixed femur
restricted by anterior
cruciate ligament

Fig. 4.5 Anatomy of the anterior cruciate ligament. (From Drake R, Vogl AW. *Gray's Anatomy for Students*. 4th ed. Philadelphia: Elsevier; 2020: Fig 6-78.)

On physical examination, patients with injury to the anterior cruciate ligament will exhibit tenderness to palpation of the anterior knee. If the ligament is avulsed from its bony insertions, tenderness may be localized to the site of insertion, whereas patients suffering from strain of the ligament have more diffuse tenderness. Patients with severe injury to the ligament may exhibit joint laxity when anterior stress is placed on the affected knee. This is best accomplished by performing an anterior drawer test for anterior cruciate ligament integrity (see Fig. 4.1). Other tests to assess the integrity of the anterior cruciate ligament include the flexion-rotation anterior drawer test and the Lachman test.

Because pain may produce muscle guarding, MRI of the knee may be necessary to confirm the clinical impression (Fig. 4.8). Joint effusion and swelling may

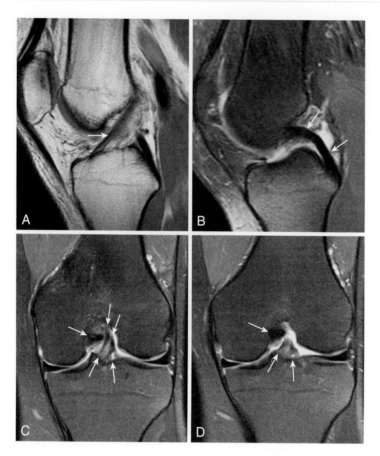

Fig. 4.6 Normal magnetic resonance imaging anatomy of the cruciate ligaments. (A) Sagittal fast spin-echo proton density (FSE PD)—weighted image shows streaky areas of isointense signal within a normal anterior cruciate ligament (ACL). Note the straight anterior border of the ACL *(arrow)*, which is parallel to Blumensaat line. (B) Sagittal fat-saturated FSE PD—weighted image shows the dark signal intensity of the posterior cruciate ligament (PCL), which has a posterior convex configuration *(arrows)*. (C, D) Contiguous coronal fat-saturated FSE PD—weighted images of a normal ACL and PCL. Note the dark signal intensity of the PCL *(arrowhead)* and relatively high signal intensity of the ACL near its tibial insertion. The anteromedial and posterolateral bundles of the ACL are visualized *(arrows)*. (From Waldman SD, Campbell RSD. *Imaging of Pain*. Philadelphia: Elsevier; 2011.)

be present with injury to the ligament, but these findings can also be suggestive of meniscal damage. Again, MRI can confirm the diagnosis.

TESTING

MRI and ultrasound imaging are indicated in all patients who present with anterior cruciate ligament injury, both to rule out coexistent internal derangement,

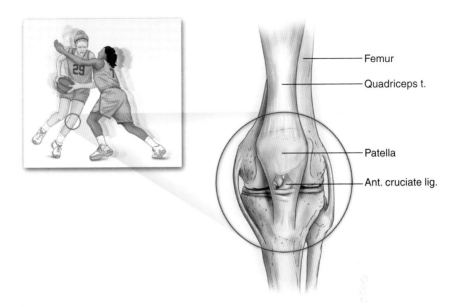

Femur

Quadriceps t.

Patella

Ant. cruciate lig.

Fig. 4.7 Anterior cruciate ligament syndrome is characterized by pain in the anterior aspect of the knee joint. It is usually the result of trauma to the anterior cruciate ligament from sudden deceleration due to the planting of the affected lower extremity while extreme twisting or hyperextension forces are placed on the knee, typically during snow skiing accidents, football, and basketball injuries. (From Waldman SD. *Atlas of Common Pain Syndromes*. 4th ed. Philadelphia: Elsevier; 2019: Fig. 109.1.)

occult mass, or tumor and to confirm the diagnosis (Figs. 4.9 and 4.10). In addition, MRI should be performed on all patients with injury to the anterior cruciate ligament who fail to respond to conservative therapy or who exhibit joint instability on clinical examination (Fig. 4.11). Bone scan may be useful to identify occult stress fractures involving the joint, especially if trauma has occurred. Based on the patient's clinical presentation, additional testing may be warranted, including a complete blood count, erythrocyte sedimentation rate, and antinuclear antibody testing.

DIFFERENTIAL DIAGNOSIS

Any condition affecting the medial compartment of the knee joint may mimic the pain of anterior cruciate ligament syndrome. Bursitis, arthritis, and entrapment neuropathies may also confuse the diagnosis, as may primary tumors of the knee and spine.

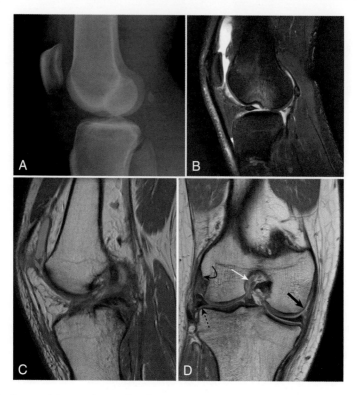

Fig. 4.8 Acute complete anterior cruciate ligament (ACL) rupture. (A) Lateral radiograph shows an impaction fracture of the lateral femoral condyle. (B) The fracture is clearly seen on the sagittal T2-weighted with fat suppression (FST2W) magnetic resonance (MR) image, with associated trabecular bone bruising in the lateral femoral condyle and a large joint effusion. (C) On the sagittal proton density (PD) MR image, there is nonvisualization of the ligament. (D) The coronal PD image demonstrates the "empty notch" sign *(white arrow)*. There is also a lateral meniscal tear *(broken black arrow)*, a partial tear of the lateral collateral ligament *(curved black arrow)*, and a grade II tear of the medial collateral ligament (MCL), including disruption of the meniscofemoral component of the deep fibers of the MCL *(black arrow)*. (From Waldman SD, Campbell RSD. *Imaging of Pain*. Philadelphia: Elsevier; 2011.)

TREATMENT

Initial treatment of the pain and functional disability associated with injury to the anterior cruciate ligament includes a combination of nonsteroidal antiinflammatory drugs or cyclooxygenase-2 inhibitors and physical therapy. The local application of heat and cold may also be beneficial. Any repetitive activity that exacerbates the patient's symptoms should be avoided. For patients who do not respond to these treatment modalities and do not have lesions that require surgical repair, injection is a reasonable next step. Injection to treat anterior cruciate

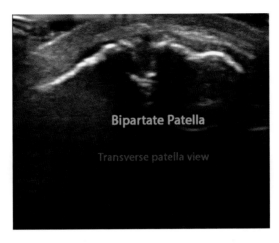

Fig. 4.9 Transverse ultrasound image of a patient with anterior knee pain demonstrating a bipartate patella. (Courtesy Steven Waldman, MD.)

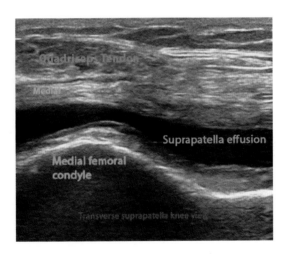

Fig. 4.10 Transverse ultrasound image demonstrating a suprapatellar effusion in a patient with an acute knee injury. (Courtesy Steven Waldman, MD.)

ligament syndrome is carried out by injecting the interarticular space of the affected knee with local anesthetic and steroid (Fig. 4.12). Ultrasound guidance may increase the accuracy of needle placement. This technique may also be used to inject platelet-rich plasma.

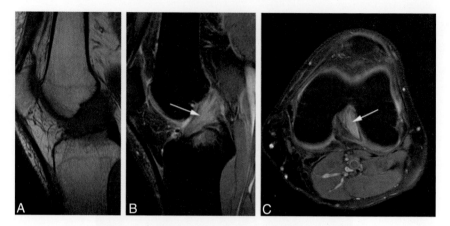

Fig. 4.11 Complete rupture of the anterior cruciate ligament. Magentic resonance image (MRI): T1-weighted sagittal views (A), proton density (PD) fat saturation (B), and PD fat saturation axial view (C). Acute ACL injury causing severe edema of the ligament, which is hypointense on T1-weighted imaging and obviously hyperintense on PD images with fat saturation *(arrows)*. (From Faruch-Bilfeld M, Lapegue F, Chiavassa H, et al. Imaging of meniscus and ligament injuries of the knee. *Diagn Interv Imaging.* 2016;97(7–8):749–765, Fig. 16.)

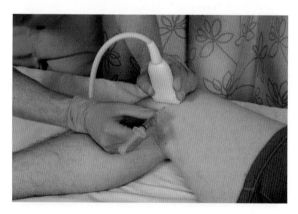

Fig. 4.12 Ultrasound-guided intraarticular injection of the knee. (Courtesy Steven Waldman, MD.)

Physical modalities, including local heat and gentle range of motion exercises, should be introduced several days after the patient undergoes injection. Vigorous exercises should be avoided because they will exacerbate the patient's symptoms. Orthotic devices to stabilize the knee may also help improve the patient's functional ability as well as pain.

HIGH-YIELD TAKEAWAYS

- The patient is afebrile, making an acute infectious etiology (e.g., septic arthritis, bursitis, or osteomyelitis) unlikely.
- The patient's symptomatology is the likely result of acute trauma to the anterior cruciate ligament.
- Since knee pain is a clinical diagnosis, physical examination and testing should be focused on not only the identification of ligamentous injury, acute arthritis, tendinitis, and bursitis, but on other pathologic processes that have the potential to harm the patient (e.g., osteomyelitis, osseous tumors, sarcomas).
- The patient heard an audible pop at the time of knee injury, suggestive of ligamentous or tendon rupture.
- The warmth and swelling of the area overlying the anterior knee is suggestive of an inflammatory process.
- The patient's symptoms are unilateral and only involve one joint, which is more suggestive of a local process than a systemic polyarthropathy.
- Plain radiographs will provide high-yield information regarding the bony contents of the joint and the identification of fractures or other bony abnormalities of the knee as well as calcification of the bursa and tendons, but ultrasound imaging and MRI will be more useful in identifying soft tissue pathology.

Suggested Readings

Lee SH, Yun SJ. Diagnosis of simultaneous acute ruptures of the anterior cruciate ligament and posterior cruciate ligament using point-of-care ultrasound in the emergency department. *J Emerg Med.* 2018;54(3):335–338, ISSN 0736-4679. Available from: https://doi.org/10.1016/j.jemermed.2017.11.014

Waldman SD. Arthritis and other abnormalities of the knee. In: *Waldman's Comprehensive Atlas of Diagnostic Ultrasound of Painful Conditions.* 1st ed. Philadelphia: Wolters Kluwer; 2016:725–740.

Waldman SD. Functional anatomy of the knee. In: *Pain Review.* 2nd ed. Philadelphia: Elsevier; 2014:142–144.

Waldman SD. Intra-articular injection of the knee. In: *Atlas of Pain Management Injection Techniques.* 4th ed. Philadelphia: Elsevier; 2014:487–490.

Waldman SD, Campbell RS, eds. Anterior cruciate ligament tear. In: *Imaging of Pain.* 1st ed. Philadelphia: Saunders; 2011:375–378.

Lincoln Mayhew

A 25-Year-Old Male With Right Anteroinferior Knee Pain and Swelling

- Learn the common causes of knee pain.
- Develop an understanding of the unique anatomy of the knee joint.
- Develop an understanding of the bursae of the knee.
- Develop an understanding of the ligaments of the knee.
- Develop an understanding of the tendons of the knee.
- Develop an understanding of the differential diagnosis of knee pain.
- Learn the clinical presentation of jumper's knee.
- Learn how to examine the knee and associated ligaments.
- Learn how to use physical examination to identify jumper's knee.
- Develop an understanding of the treatment options for jumper's knee.

Lincoln Mayhew

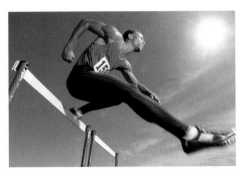

Lincoln Mayhew is a 25-year-old male track star with the chief complaint of "my right knee keeps swelling up and hurting." Lincoln stated that over the past few weeks, his right knee has become increasingly swollen and painful, especially after his workout. "Doc, as an elite athlete, I have to stay in shape—you know, sprints, hurdles, and laps. I can't miss a day." Lincoln noted that he was competing in a regional qualifier and he landed "kind of funny" on his right knee. His knee was a little sore that night, but he thought he would just work through it, so he didn't alter his routine. He tried the whirlpool, analgesic balm, an elastic wrap, and Motrin, but in spite of all this, his knee pain got worse and it started to swell.

"Doctor, I've got to get my knee better. Can you just give me a shot or something? I have a big meet coming up and I don't know how I can compete like this." I asked Lincoln about any previous injuries to the right knee and he said that both of his knees could be sore after a heavy workout, but he had never had anything like this.

I asked Lincoln what made his symptoms worse and he said, "Anytime I put weight on my right knee, I'm in trouble. I have trouble walking, and have been sleeping on the couch because it's so hard trying to walk upstairs to my bedroom. Between the couch and the knee pain, my sleep is really off."

I asked Lincoln to point with one finger to show me where the pain was and he pointed to the area in front of his right knee just below the patella and said, "It hurts right here, Doc."

On physical examination, Lincoln was afebrile. His respirations were 16 and his pulse was 65 and regular. His blood pressure was 120/70. Lincoln's head, eys, ears, nose, and throat (HEENT) exam was normal, as was his cardiopulmonary examination. His thyroid was normal, as was his abdominal examination. There was no costovertebral angle (CVA) tenderness. There was no peripheral edema. His low back examination was unremarkable. Visual inspection of the right knee revealed a large effusion, which I confirmed with the ballottement test (see Fig. 2.2). The area over the anterior knee was warm but did not appear to be infected. There was significant tenderness with palpation of the superior and inferior poles of the patella as well as with palpation of the patellar tendon (Fig. 5.1). Examination of the bursae of the knee revealed no obvious bursitis, but the swelling of the knee could have hidden subtle findings. I performed the single-leg decline squat test, which was markedly positive on the right and

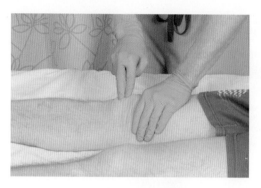

Fig. 5.1   Patients suffering from jumper's knee often have large joint effusions and exhibit a positive ballottement test. To perform the ballottement test for knee effusions, the clinician has the patient extend
and fully relax the knee. The clinician then grasps the affected knee just above the joint space and applies
pressure to displace synovial fluid from the suprapatellar pouch into the joint, which will elevate the patella.
The clinician then ballotes the patella. The test is considered positive if the patella ballotes easily. (From
Waldman SD. *Atlas of Common Pain Syndromes*. 4th ed. Philadelphia: Elsevier; 2019: Fig. 110.3.)

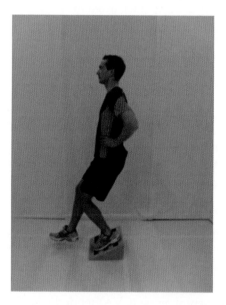

Fig. 5.2   The single-leg decline squat test. (From Rudavsky A, Cook J. Physiotherapy management of
patellar tendinopathy [jumper's knee]. *J Physiother*. 2014;60[3]:122–129, Fig. 2.)

negative on the left (Fig. 5.2). Range of motion of the knee joint, especially
resisted extension of the joint, reproduced Lincoln's pain. The left knee examination was normal, as was examination of his other major joints. A careful neurologic examination of the upper and lower extremities revealed that there was no
evidence of peripheral or entrapment neuropathy, and the deep tendon reflexes
were normal.

Key Clinical Points—What's Important and What's Not

THE HISTORY

- Onset of right knee pain and swelling of the right knee following landing wrong after jumping a hurdle
- Significant swelling of the right knee
- Pain localized to the anterior knee
- Difficulty walking stairs
- No other specific traumatic event to the area identified
- No fever or chills
- Sleep disturbance

THE PHYSICAL EXAMINATION

- The patient is afebrile
- There is no ecchymosis over the anterior knee
- There is significant swelling of the knee
- Tenderness to palpation of the patellar tendon on the right
- Tenderness to palpation of the superior and inferior poles of the patella on the right
- No evidence of infection
- Pain on resisted extension of the affected right knee
- The single-leg decline squat test was positive on the right (see Fig. 5.2)

OTHER FINDINGS OF NOTE

- Normal HEENT examination
- Normal cardiovascular examination
- Normal pulmonary examination
- Normal abdominal examination
- No peripheral edema
- Normal upper and lower extremity neurologic examination, motor and sensory examination
- No evidence of bursitis
- Examinations of other joints other than the right knee were normal

What Tests Would You Like to Order?

The following tests were ordered:
- Plain radiographs of the right knee
- Ultrasound of the right knee
- Magnetic resonance imaging (MRI) of the right knee

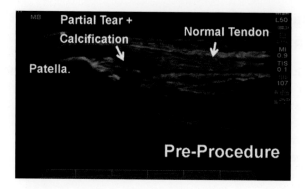

Fig. 5.3 The patellar tendon is readily visualized by ultrasound as it attaches to the inferior pole of the patella. The normal tendon appears as a homogeneous, discrete linear image. The ultrasonic image of tendinopathy is that of a hypoechoic region that is a dark or black area within the substance of the involved tendon. (From Elattrache NS, Morrey BF. Percutaneous ultrasonic tenotomy as a treatment for chronic patellar tendinopathy—jumper's knee. *Oper Tech Orthop*. 2013;23(2):98–103, Fig. 2.)

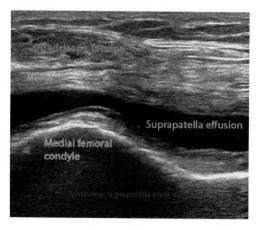

Fig. 5.4 Transverse ultrasound image demonstrating a large joint effusion spreading to the suprapatellar area. (Courtesy Steven Waldman, MD.)

TEST RESULTS

The plain radiographs of the right knee were reported as normal. Ultrasound examination of the right knee revealed tendinopathy of the patellar tendon and a large joint effusion (Figs. 5.3 and 5.4). MRI examination of the right knee demonstrates significant patellar tendinopathy consistent with jumper's knee (Fig. 5.5).

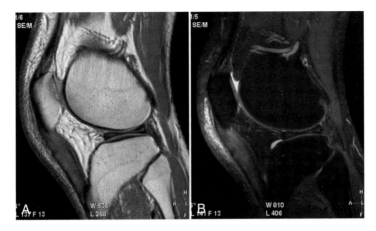

Fig. 5.5 Sagittal T1W (A) and fat-suppressed T2-weighted (FST2W) (B) magnetic resonance (MR) images of a patient with diffuse patellar tendinopathy. The tendon is thickened and of increased signal intensity (SI) on both pulse sequences, but the SI is not as bright as that of fluid on the FST2W MR image. High-SI prepatellar bursitis is also evident on the FST2W MR image. (From Waldman SD, Campbell RSD. *Imaging of Pain*. Philadelphia: Elsevier; 2011.)

📋 Clinical Correlation—Putting It All Together

What is the diagnosis?
- Jumper's knee

The Science Behind the Diagnosis
ANATOMY

The quadriceps tendon is made up of fibers from the four muscles that comprise the quadriceps muscle: the vastus lateralis, the vastus intermedius, the vastus medialis, and the rectus femoris (Fig. 5.6). These muscles are the primary extensors for lower extremity at the knee. The tendons of these muscles converge and unite to form a single, exceedingly strong tendon. The patella functions as a sesamoid bone within the quadriceps tendon, with fibers for tendon expanding around the patella and forming the medial and lateral patella retinacula, which help strengthen the knee joint. These fibers are called expansions and are subject to strain; the tendon proper is subject to the development of tendinitis (Fig. 5.7). These fibers continue as the patellar tendon, which originates at the superior pole of the patella and is comprised of fibers from the quadriceps tendon. The fibers pass over the top of and on each side of the patella to ultimately insert on

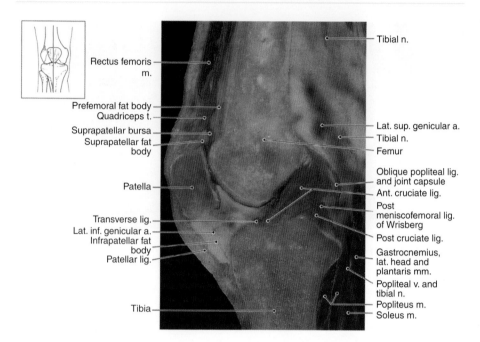

Fig. 5.6 Sagittal view of the knee. (From Waldman SD. *Atlas of Common Pain Syndromes*. 4th ed. Philadelphia: Elsevier; 2019: Fig. 110.2.)

the tibial tuberosity. The suprapatellar, infrapatellar, and prepatellar bursae also may concurrently become inflamed with dysfunction of the quadriceps and patellar tendons.

CLINICAL SYNDROME

The patellar tendon, which is also known as the patellar ligament, originates at the superior pole of the patella and is comprised of fibers from the quadriceps tendon, which pass over the top of and on each side of the patella to ultimately insert on the tibial tuberosity (see Fig. 5.7). The fibers of the patellar tendon are susceptible to strain or sprain as the result of overuse or misuse of the knee, as is seen in long-distance running or from direct trauma to the quadriceps tendon and patella from kicks or head butts. A distinct clinical entity from tendonitis of the patellar tendon, jumper's knee is a tendinopathy resulting from a repetitive stress disorder that is thought to be the result of the strong eccentric contraction of the quadriceps muscle that is necessary to strengthen the knee joint during landing rather than from the jump itself (Fig. 5.8). Tendinitis of the quadriceps or patellar tendons or quadriceps

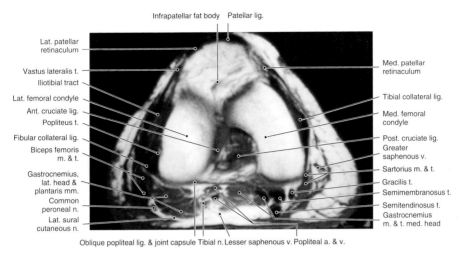

Infrapatellar fat body   Patellar lig.

Lat. patellar retinaculum

Vastus lateralis t.
Iliotibial tract
Lat. femoral condyle
Ant. cruciate lig.
Popliteus t.
Fibular collateral lig.
Biceps femoris m. & t.
Gastrocnemius, lat. head & plantaris mm.
Common peroneal n.
Lat. sural cutaneous n.

Med. patellar retinaculum

Tibial collateral lig.
Med. femoral condyle

Post. cruciate lig.
Greater saphenous v.
Sartorius m. & t.
Gracilis t.
Semimembranosus t.
Semitendinosus t.
Gastrocnemius m. & t. med. head

Oblique popliteal lig. & joint capsule Tibial n. Lesser saphenous v. Popliteal a. & v.

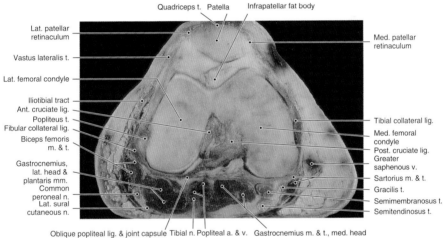

Quadriceps t.   Patella   Infrapatellar fat body

Lat. patellar retinaculum

Vastus lateralis t.

Lat. femoral condyle

Iliotibial tract
Ant. cruciate lig.
Popliteus t.
Fibular collateral lig.
Biceps femoris m. & t.
Gastrocnemius, lat. head & plantaris mm.
Common peroneal n.
Lat. sural cutaneous n.

Med. patellar retinaculum

Tibial collateral lig.
Med. femoral condyle
Post. cruciate lig.
Greater saphenous v.
Sartorius m. & t.
Gracilis t.
Semimembranosus t.
Semitendinosus t.

Oblique popliteal lig. & joint capsule Tibial n. Popliteal a. & v.   Gastrocnemius m. & t., med. head

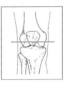

Fig. 5.7 The patella functions as a sesamoid bone within the quadriceps tendon, with fibers for tendon expanding around the patella and forming the medial and lateral patella retinacula, which help strengthen the knee joint. (From Waldman SD. *Atlas of Pain Management Injection Techniques*. 4th ed. St Louis: Elsevier; 2017: Fig. 138-4.)

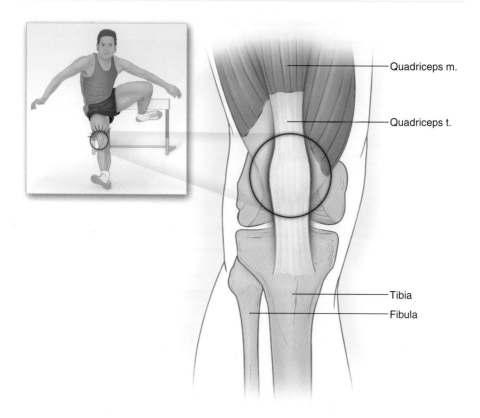

Quadriceps m.

Quadriceps t.

Tibia
Fibula

Fig. 5.8 Jumper's knee—characterized by pain at the inferior or superior pole of the patella—occurs in up to 20% of jumping athletes at some point in their careers. (From Waldman SD. *Atlas of Common Pain Syndromes*. 4th ed. Philadelphia: Elsevier; 2019: Fig 110.1.)

expansion syndrome may coexist with jumper's knee and confuse the clinical picture. Congenital variants of the anatomy of the knee such as bipartite patella, patella alta or baja, and limb length discrepancies, as well as weak or poor quadriceps and hamstring muscle flexibility, have been implicated as risk factors for the development of jumper's knee (Fig. 5.9).

SIGNS AND SYMPTOMS

Patients suffering from jumper's knee will complain of pain over the superior and/or inferior poles of the patella. Unlike quadriceps expansion syndrome, which has a predilection for the medial side of the patella, jumper's knee can afflict both the medial and lateral tendon fibers. Frequently, the patient suffering from jumper's knee will bitterly complain of increased pain when walking down

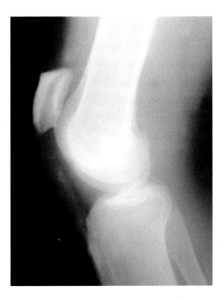

Fig. 5.9 Congenital variants of the anatomy of the knee such as bipartite patella, patella alta or baja, and limb length discrepancies as well as weak or poor quadriceps and hamstring muscle flexibility have been implicated as risk factors for the development of jumper's knee.

stairs or slopes, especially on uneven surfaces as when hiking. The pain is constant and is characterized as aching with activity exacerbating the pain. The pain of jumper's knee injury may interfere with sleep. On physical examination, there is tenderness of the quadriceps and/or patellar tendons. A joint effusion may be appreciated on ballottement of the patella (see Fig. 2.2). Active resisted extension of the knee reproduces the pain. Coexistent suprapatellar and infrapatellar bursitis, tendinitis, arthritis, or internal derangement for knee may confuse the clinical picture after trauma to the knee joint.

TESTING

Plain radiographs are indicated in all patients who present with knee pain (Fig. 5.10). MRI of the knee is indicated if jumper's knee is suspected because it readily demonstrates tendinosis of the quadriceps or patellar tendon (see Fig. 5.5). Ultrasound imaging may also provide beneficial information regarding the vascularity and integrity of the patellar and quadriceps tendons and patellar retinacula (Fig. 5.11). Bone scan may be useful to identify occult stress fractures involving the joint, especially if trauma has occurred. Based on the patient's clinical presentation, additional testing may be indicated, including a complete blood count, erythrocyte sedimentation rate, and antinuclear antibody testing.

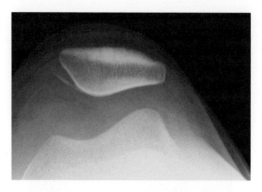

Fig. 5.10 Merchant view of patella, showing lateral patellar subluxation, increased patellar tilt, and a bone fragment from the medial edge corresponding to medial patellofemoral ligament (MPFL) avulsion. (From Duthon VB. Acute traumatic patellar dislocation. *Orthop Traumatol Surgery Res*. 2015;101(1): S59—S67, Fig. 6.)

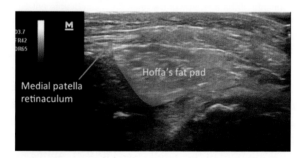

Fig. 5.11 Ultrasound image demonstrating the medial patellar retinaculum and Hoffa fat pad. (Courtesy Steven Waldman, MD.)

DIFFERENTIAL DIAGNOSIS

Jumper's knee is a repetitive stress disorder that causes tendinosis of the quadriceps and patellar tendons and is a distinct clinical entity from tendinitis of those tendons or quadriceps expansion syndrome, which may coexist with jumper's knee and confuse the clinical picture. Quadriceps expansion syndrome has a predilection for the medial side of the superior pole of the patella. The quadriceps tendon is also subject to acute calcific tendinitis, which may coexist with acute strain injuries and the more chronic changes of jumper's knee. Calcific tendinitis of the quadriceps has a characteristic radiographic appearance of whiskers on the anterosuperior patella. The suprapatellar, infrapatellar, and prepatellar bursae also may become inflamed with dysfunction of the quadriceps tendon.

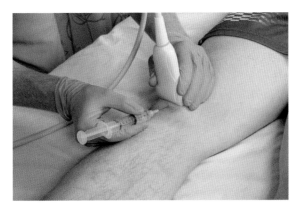

Fig. 5.12 Ultrasound-guided injection of the patellar tendon. (Courtesy Steven Waldman, MD.)

TREATMENT

Initial treatment of the pain and functional disability associated with jumper's knee includes a combination of nonsteroidal antiinflammatory drugs (NSAIDs) or cyclooxygenase-2 inhibitors and physical therapy. A nighttime splint to protect the knee may also help relieve the symptoms. For patients who do not respond to these treatment modalities, injection with local anesthetic and steroid is a reasonable next step (Fig. 5.12).

Physical modalities, including local heat and gentle range of motion exercises, should be introduced several days after the patient undergoes injection. Vigorous exercises should be avoided because they will exacerbate the patient's symptoms. Simple analgesics and NSAIDs can be used concurrently with this injection technique. Recent reports suggest that the injection of platelet-rich plasma may aid in the healing of the tendinopathy associated with jumper's knee.

HIGH-YIELD TAKEAWAYS

- The patient is afebrile, making an acute infectious etiology (e.g., septic arthritis, bursitis, or osteomyelitis) unlikely.
- The patient's symptomatology is the likely result of chronic overuse and irritation of the patellar tendon.
- Since knee pain is a clinical diagnosis, physical examination and testing should be focused on not only the identification of ligamentous injury, acute arthritis, tendinitis, and bursitis, but on other pathologic processes that have the potential to harm the patient (e.g., osteomyelitis, osseous tumors, sarcomas).

(Continued)

- Warmth and swelling of the knee suggest an inflammatory process.
- The patient's symptoms are unilateral and involve only one joint, which is more suggestive of a local process than a systemic polyarthropathy.
- Plain radiographs will provide high-yield information regarding the bony contents of the joint and the identification of fractures or other bony abnormalities of the knee as well as calcification of the bursa and tendons, but ultrasound imaging and MRI will be more useful in identifying soft tissue pathology.

Suggested Readings

Abdelbary MH, Bassiouny A. Ultrasound guided injection in patellar tendinopathy; clinical outcomes of platelet-rich plasma compared to high-volume injection. *Egypt J Radiol Nuclear Med*. 2018;543—547.

Basas A, Cook J, Gómez MA, et al. Effects of a strength protocol combined with electrical stimulation on patellar tendinopathy: 42 months retrospective follow-up on 6 high-level jumping athletes. *Phys Ther Sport*. 2018;34:105—112.

Elattrache NS, Morrey BF. Percutaneous ultrasonic tenotomy as a treatment for chronic patellar tendinopathy—jumper's knee. *Oper Tech Orthop*. 2013;23(2):98—103.

Lueders DR, Smith J, Sellon JL. Ultrasound-guided knee procedures. *Phys Med Rehab Clin N Am*. 2016;27(3):631—648.

Pascarella F, Giuseppe Di Salvatore M, Pezzella R, et al. Arthroscopic treatment of jumper's knee in professional athletes. *Revue de Chirurgie Orthopédique et Traumatologique*. 2017;103(8):S267—S268.

Rudavsky A, Cook J. Physiotherapy management of patellar tendinopathy (jumper's knee). *J Physiother*. 2014;60(3):122—129.

Waldman SD. Arthritis and other abnormalities of the knee. In: *Waldman's Comprehensive Atlas of Diagnostic Ultrasound of Painful Conditions*. 1st ed. Philadelphia: Wolters Kluwer; 2016:725—750.

Waldman SD. Functional Anatomy of the Knee. In: *Pain Review*. 2nd ed. Philadelphia: Elsevier; 2015:152—155.

Waldman SD. Jumper's knee. In: *Atlas of Common Pain Syndromes*. 4h ed. Philadelphia: Elsevier; 2019:435—439.

Waldman SD. Jumper's knee and other abnormalities of the patella. In: *Waldman's Comprehensive Atlas of Diagnostic Ultrasound of Painful Conditions*. 1st ed. Philadelphia: Wolters Kluwer; 2016:771—779.

Waldman SD, Campbell RSD. Anatomy, special imaging considerations for knee. *Imaging of Pain*. 1st ed. Philadelphia: Saunders Elsevier; 2011:367—368.

Mike Montgomery

A 26-Year-Old Male Long-Distance Runner With Right Lateral Knee Pain

- Learn the common causes of knee pain.
- Develop an understanding of the unique anatomy of the knee joint.
- Develop an understanding of the bursae of the knee.
- Develop an understanding of the ligaments of the knee.
- Develop an understanding of the tendons of the knee.
- Develop an understanding of the differential diagnosis of knee pain.
- Learn the clinical presentation of runner's knee.
- Learn how to examine the knee and associated ligaments.
- Learn how to use physical examination to identify runner's knee.
- Develop an understanding of the treatment options for runner's knee.

Mike Montgomery

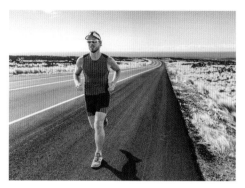

Mike Montgomery is a 26-year-old male long-distance runner with the chief complaint of, "My right knee is killing me." Mike stated that he just got back from running an Iron Man triathlon in Hawaii. "Doc, it was a rough one this time. Between the rain and the humidity, it was really a challenge—even for me. A lot of the course was wet and there was a fair amount of mud, so I was really slipping around. The unsteady footing was really hard on my knees. Since I got back, I can barely walk because the outside of my knee hurts so much. I keep looking at it expecting a big bruise, but there's nothing to look at. I can barely touch it, though, because it hurts so bad." Mike said that he tried resting the knee, using the hot tub at the gym, Icy Hot, an Ace wrap, and Advil, but in spite of all of this, his knee just hadn't improved. If anything, it was a little worse.

"Doc, I've really got to get my knee better. I deliver for UPS and if I can't get in and out of the truck and carry packages up to the door, I am screwed." I asked Mike about any previous injuries to the right knee and he said that both of his knees could be sore after a long run, but he had never had anything like this.

I asked Mike what made his symptoms worse and he said, "Anytime I put weight on my right knee, I'm in trouble. Like I said, I can barely walk, and stairs are a real pistol. My sleep is completely jacked up because of the knee pain and worry."

I asked Mike to point with one finger to show me where the pain was and he pointed to a point over the lateral epicondyle of the femur. "X marks the spot. It's right here!" I asked if the pain radiated anywhere else and Mike just shook his head.

On physical examination, Mike was afebrile. His respirations were 16 and his pulse was 62 and regular. His blood pressure was 118/68. Mike's head, eyes, ears, nose, and throat (HEENT) exam was normal, as was his cardiopulmonary examination. His thyroid was normal, as was his abdominal examination. There was no costovertebral angle (CVA) tenderness. There was no peripheral edema. His low back examination was unremarkable. Visual inspection of the right knee revealed no evidence of ecchymosis or swelling. The area over the right lateral knee was warm but did not appear to be infected. There was significant point tenderness over the lateral epicondyle of the femur. Examination of the bursae of the knee revealed no obvious bursitis,

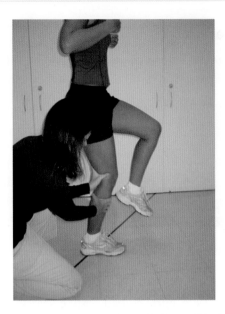

Fig. 6.1 The modified Noble compression test. (From Waldman SD. *Atlas of Pain Management Injection Techniques*. 4th ed. St Louis: Elsevier; 2017: Fig. 147-3.)

but a subtle iliotibial bursitis could be hard to identify given the amount of pain elicited when palpating the area.

Range of motion of the knee joint and resisted abduction of the joint reproduced Mike's pain. A modified Noble compression test was positive on the right (Fig. 6.1). The left knee examination was normal, as was examination of his other major joints. A careful neurologic examination of the upper and lower extremities revealed there was no evidence of peripheral or entrapment neuropathy, and the deep tendon reflexes were normal.

Key Clinical Points—What's Important and What's Not

THE HISTORY

- Onset of right lateral knee pain following completing an Iron Man triathalon
- Significant pain on ambulation
- Pain localized to the lateral knee
- Difficulty walking stairs
- No other specific traumatic event to the area identified
- No fever or chills
- Sleep disturbance

THE PHYSICAL EXAMINATION

- The patient is afebrile
- There is no ecchymosis over the lateral knee
- There is significant swelling of the knee
- Point tenderness over the lateral epicondyle of the right femur
- No evidence of infection
- Pain on resisted abduction of the affected lower extremity
- The modified Noble compression test was positive on the right (see Fig. 6.1)

OTHER FINDINGS OF NOTE

- Normal HEENT examination
- Normal cardiovascular examination
- Normal pulmonary examination
- Normal abdominal examination
- No peripheral edema
- Normal upper and lower extremity neurologic examination, motor and sensory examination
- No evidence of bursitis
- Examinations of other joints other than the right knee were normal

 ## What Tests Would You Like to Order?

The following tests were ordered:
- Plain radiographs of the right knee
- Ultrasound of the right knee
- Magnetic resonance imaging (MRI) of the right knee

TEST RESULTS

The plain radiographs of the right knee were reported as normal. Ultrasound examination of the right knee revealed edematous swelling of the soft tissues deep to the iliotibial band (Fig. 6.2). MRI examination of the right knee demonstrates high intensity signal deep to the iliotibial tract consistent with runner's knee (Fig. 6.3).

 ## Clinical Correlation—Putting It All Together

What is the diagnosis?
- Runner's knee

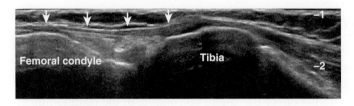

Fig. 6.2 Iliotibial band syndrome. Wide longitudinal ultrasound scan along the iliotibial band *(arrows):* edematous swelling of the soft tissues deep to the iliotibial band, whose fibers do not show any alteration. (From Draghi F, Danesino GM, Coscia D, et al. Overload syndromes of the knee in adolescents: sonographic findings. *J Ultrasound* 2008;11:151–157.)

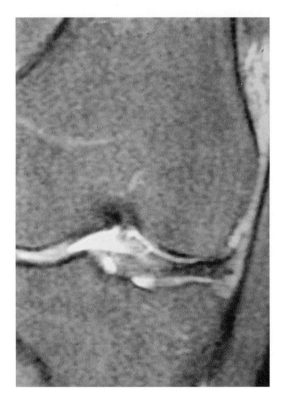

Fig. 6.3 Iliotibial tract syndrome: magnetic resonance (MR) imaging. This coronal fat-suppressed fast spin-echo (TR/TE, 2500/42) MR image shows an abnormal, poorly defined region of high signal intensity deep to the iliotibial tract. (From Resnick D. *Diagnosis of Bone and Joint Disorders*. 4th ed. Philadelphia: Saunders; 2002.)

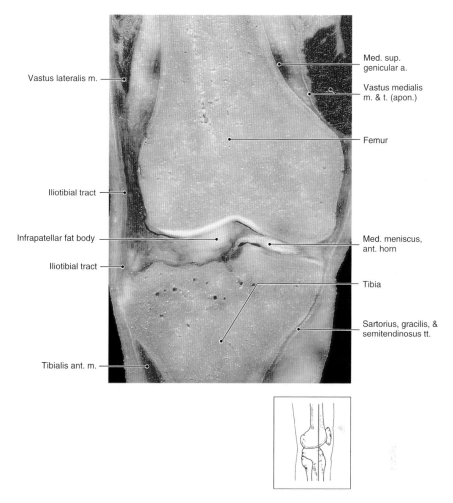

Fig. 6.4 Anatomy of the iliotibial tract and adjacent structures. *apon.*, Aponeurosis; *m.*, muscle; *med.*, medial; *sup.*, superior; *t./tt.*, tendon/tendons. (From Kang HS, Ahn JM, Resnick D. *MRI of the Extremities: An Anatomic Atlas*. 2nd ed. Philadelphia: Saunders; 2002.)

The Science Behind the Diagnosis

ANATOMY

The iliotibial band bursa lies between the iliotibial band and the lateral condyle of the femur. The iliotibial band is an extension of the fascia lata, which inserts at the lateral condyle of the tibia (Figs. 6.4 and 6.5). The iliotibial band can rub backward and forward over the lateral epicondyle of the femur and become

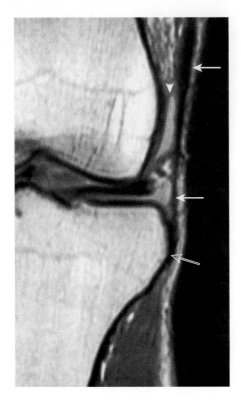

Fig. 6.5 Normal iliotibial tract: magnetic resonance (MR) imaging. A coronal intermediate-weighted (TR/TE, 2000/20) spin-echo MR image shows the iliotibial tract *(solid arrows)* attaching to the Gerdy tubercle *(open arrow)* in the tibia. A small joint effusion is evident just medial to the iliotibial tract *(arrowhead)*. (From Resnick D. *Diagnosis of Bone and Joint Disorders*. 4th ed. Philadelphia: Saunders; 2002.)

inflamed (Fig. 6.6). This rubbing can also irritate the iliotibial bursa beneath it. The iliotibial bursa is subject to the development of inflammation caused by overuse, misuse, or direct trauma.

CLINICAL SYNDROME

Runner's knee is a relatively uncommon cause of lateral knee pain encountered in clinical practice. Also known as *iliotibial band friction syndrome*, runner's knee is an overuse syndrome caused by friction injury to the iliotibial band as it rubs back and forth across the lateral epicondyle of the femur during running (Fig. 6.7). Runner's knee is a clinical entity distinct from iliotibial bursitis, although these two painful conditions frequently coexist. This painful

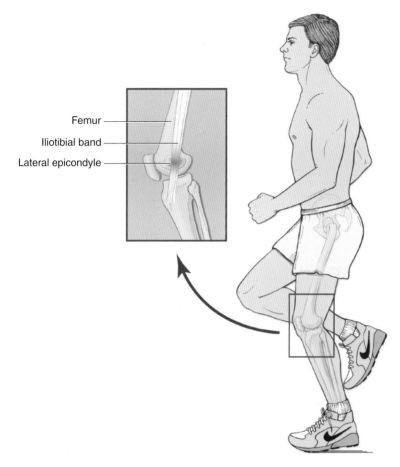

Femur
Iliotibial band
Lateral epicondyle

Fig. 6.6 Pathophysiology of iliotibial band syndrome. (From Waldman SD. *Atlas of Pain Management Injection Techniques*. 4th ed. St Louis: Elsevier; 2007: Fig. 147-1.)

condition occurs more commonly in patients with genu varum and planus feet, although worn-out jogging shoes also have been implicated in the evolution of this disease.

SIGNS AND SYMPTOMS

Physical examination may reveal point tenderness over the lateral epicondyle of the femur just above the tendinous insertion of the iliotibial band. If coexistent iliotibial bursitis is present, swelling and fluid accumulation that surrounds the bursa often are present (Fig. 6.8). Palpation of this area while

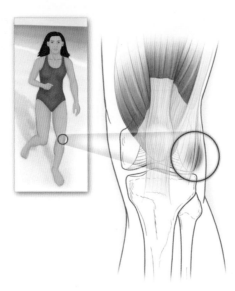

Fig. 6.7 Also known as iliotibial band friction syndrome, runner's knee is an overuse syndrome caused by friction injury to the iliotibial band as it rubs back and forth across the lateral epicondyle of the femur during running. (From Waldman SD. *Atlas of Uncommon Pain Syndromes*. 4th ed. Philadelphia: Saunders; 2020: Fig. 117-1.)

having the patient flex and extend the knee may result in a creaking or "catching" sensation. Active resisted abduction of the lower extremity and passive adduction reproduce the pain. Sudden release of resistance during this maneuver markedly increases the pain. Pain is exacerbated by having the patient stand with all the weight on the affected extremity and then flexing the affected knee 30 to 40 degrees.

TESTING

Plain radiographs of the knee may reveal calcification of the bursa and associated structures, including the iliotibial band tendon, consistent with chronic inflammation. MRI and ultrasound are indicated if runner's knee, iliotibial band bursitis, internal derangement, occult mass, or tumor of the knee is suspected (Figs. 6.9 and 6.10). Electromyography helps distinguish iliotibial band bursitis from neuropathy, lumbar radiculopathy, and plexopathy. Injection of the iliotibial band at the friction point may serve as a diagnostic and therapeutic maneuver.

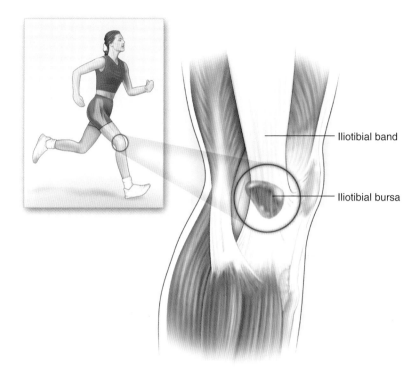

Iliotibial band

Iliotibial bursa

Fig. 6.8 The onset of iliotibial bursitis frequently occurs after long-distance cycling or jogging with worn-out shoes without proper cushioning. Flexion of the affected knee may reproduce the pain. Often, the patient is unable to kneel or walk down stairs. (From Waldman SD. *Atlas of Uncommon Pain Syndromes*. 4th ed. Philadelphia: Saunders; 2020: Fig. 120.1.)

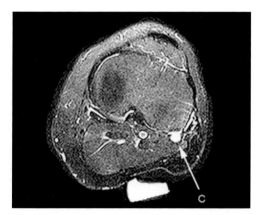

Fig. 6.9 Magnetic resonance imaging (MRI) of a patient with the clinical diagnosis of runner's knee. Fluid collection *(C)* posterior to the lateral femoral condyle is consistent with a synovial cyst with no fluid deep to the iliotibial band. (From Costa ML, Marshall T, Donell ST, et al. Knee synovial cyst presenting as iliotibial band friction syndrome. *Knee*. 2004;11[3]:247−248, Fig. 1.)

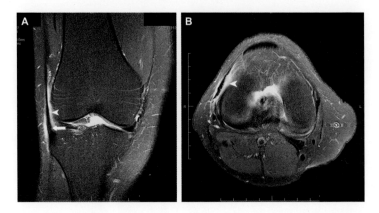

Fig 6.10 Iliotibial band friction syndrome. (A) Coronal T2 fat-saturated image demonstrates high signal intensity in the fatty tissue deep to the iliotibial band *(arrowhead)* with loss of definition of the normally low signal intensity band *(arrow)*. (B) Axial T2 fat-saturated image demonstrates high signal intensity in the fatty tissue deep to the iliotibial band, consistent with replacement by inflammatory tissue *(arrowhead)*. (From O'Keeffe SA, Hogan BA, Eustace SL, et al. Overuse injuries of the knee. *MRI Clin N Am.* 2009;17[4]:725–739, Fig. 9.)

DIFFERENTIAL DIAGNOSIS

The most common cause of lateral knee pain is degenerative arthritis of the knee. Other pathologic processes may mimic the pain and functional disability of runner's knee. Lumbar radiculopathy may cause pain and disability similar to that of runner's knee. In such patients, back pain is usually present, and the knee examination should be negative. Entrapment neuropathies of the lower extremity, such as meralgia paresthetica, and bursitis of the knee also may confuse the diagnosis; both conditions may coexist with runner's knee. Primary and metastatic tumors of the femur and proximal tibia and fibula may manifest in a manner analogous to runner's knee.

TREATMENT

Initial treatment of the pain and functional disability associated with runner's knee should include a combination of nonsteroidal antiinflammatory drugs or cyclooxygenase-2 inhibitors and physical therapy. Local application of heat and cold may be beneficial. For patients who do not respond to these treatment modalities, injection of the iliotibial band at its friction point with a local anesthetic and steroid may be a reasonable next step (Fig. 6.11).

Ultrasound guidance may increase the accuracy of needle placement and decrease the incidence of needle-related complications.

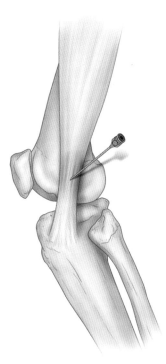

Fig. 6.11   Injection technique for runner's knee and iliotibial bursitis. (From Waldman SD. *Atlas of Pain Management Injection Techniques*. 4th ed. St Louis: Elsevier; 2017: Fig. 147-6.)

HIGH-YIELD TAKEAWAYS

- The patient is afebrile, making an acute infectious etiology (e.g., septic arthritis, bursitis, or osteomyelitis) unlikely.
- The patient's symptomatology is the likely result of chronic overuse and irritation of the iliotibial band and possibly the iliotibial bursa.
- Since knee pain is a clinical diagnosis, physical examination and testing should be focused on not only the identification of ligamentous injury, acute arthritis, tendinitis, and bursitis, but on other pathologic processes that have the potential to harm the patient (e.g., osteomyelitis, osseous tumors, sarcomas).
- Warmth of the lateral knee suggests an inflammatory process.
- The patient's symptoms are unilateral and involve only one joint, which is more suggestive of a local process than a systemic polyarthropathy.

(Continued)

- Plain radiographs will provide high-yield information regarding the bony contents of the joint and the identification of fractures or other bony abnormalities of the knee as well as calcification of the bursa and tendons, but ultrasound imaging and MRI will be more useful in identifying soft tissue pathology.

Suggested Readings

Waldman SD. Arthritis and other abnormalities of the knee. In: *Waldman's Comprehensive Atlas of Diagnostic Ultrasound of Painful Conditions*. Philadelphia: Wolters Kluwer; 2016:726–760.

Waldman SD. Functional anatomy of the knee. In: *Pain Review*. 2nd ed. Philadelphia: Elsevier; 2016:162–166.

Waldman SD. Runner's knee. In: *Atlas of Common Pain Syndromes*. 4th ed. Philadelphia: Elsevier; 2019:440–445.

Waldman SD. Injection technique to relieve pain secondary to iliotibial band bursitis. In: *Atlas of Pain Management Injection Techniques*. 4th ed. Philadelphia: Elsevier; 2017:292–294.

Waldman SD. The iliotibial band bursa. In: *Pain Review*. 2nd ed. Philadelphia: Elsevier; 2016:148–149.

Waldman SD, Campbell RSD. Anatomy, special imaging considerations for knee. In: *Imaging of Pain*. Philadelphia: Saunders Elsevier; 2011:367–368.

Andrew Kelsey

A 27-Year-Old Carpet Layer With Severe Left Knee Pain and Swelling

- Learn the common causes of knee pain.
- Develop an understanding of the unique anatomy of the knee joint.
- Develop an understanding of the bursae of the knee.
- Develop an understanding of the causes of suprapatellar bursitis.
- Develop an understanding of the differential diagnosis of suprapatellar bursitis.
- Learn the clinical presentation of suprapatellar bursitis.
- Learn how to examine the knee and associated bursae.
- Learn how to use physical examination to identify suprapatellar bursitis.
- Develop an understanding of the treatment options for suprapatellar bursitis.

Andrew Kelsey

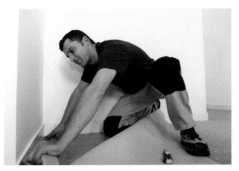

Andrew Kelsey is a 27-year-old carpet layer with the chief complaint of, "My left knee really hurts." Andrew stated that he just completed laying carpet in the new downtown convention center. "We really got behind on this project so at the end, there was a lot of overtime. At first, by the end of the day, my knee felt a little squishy and it was sore. The Motrin helped the soreness and by morning, the swelling was a little better. By the time we got the job finished, my knee was swollen 24/7 and it hurt whenever I put any weight on it. Whenever I got down on my knees or squatted, the pain went through the roof. Doc, I've got to keep working, so I need you to just give me a shot in the knee."

I asked Andrew about any antecedent knee trauma and he just shook his head no, but went on to say that from time to time, his left knee would bother him a little after a long day of "kicking in carpeting, but usually a couple of Motrin would take care of it," and he was "good to go." He also tried to use a heating pad, which he thought made it worse and made the pain go up into the front of his thigh. Andrew said that he felt the knee was kind of swollen and "squishy" and that it felt hot to touch. I asked Andrew what made his pain worse and he said, "Anytime I start to walk or whenever I squat it hurts, and over the last few days I can't kneel on my left knee. Doc, I have to put all my weight on my right knee, which is really starting to complain. And the crazy thing is, now my back is hurting from the way I'm working. I'm already tired, as my knee is keeping me up at night—or maybe it's just the worrying about my job."

I asked Andrew to point with one finger to show me where it hurt the most. He pointed to the area just above the left patella and said, "Doctor, it's right here!"

On physical examination, Andrew was afebrile. His respirations were 18 and his pulse was 76 and regular. His blood pressure was 138/78. Andrew's head, eyes, ears, nose, and throat (HEENT) exam was normal, as was his cardiopulmonary examination. His thyroid was normal. His abdominal examination revealed no abnormal mass or organomegaly. There was no costovertebral angle (CVA) tenderness. There was no peripheral edema. His low back examination revealed some tenderness to deep palpation of the paraspinous musculature. Visual inspection of the left lateral knee revealed moderate swelling. The area over the left suprapatellar area felt a little warm but did not appear to be infected. The left knee felt "boggy" on palpation, and there was marked tenderness to palpation

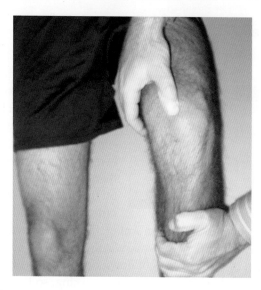

Fig. 7.1 The resisted extension release test for suprapatellar bursitis. (From Waldman SD. *Physical Diagnosis of Pain: An Atlas of Signs and Symptoms*. 3rd ed. St Louis: Elsevier; 2016: Fig. 224-3.)

over the suprapatellar region. Palpation of this area exacerbated Andrew's pain. Range of motion of the knee joint, especially resisted extension and passive flexion of the knee joint, caused Andrew to cry out in pain. I performed a resisted extension release test, which was markedly positive on the left and negative on the right (Fig. 7.1). The right knee examination was normal, as was examination of his major joints. A careful neurologic examination of the upper and lower extremities revealed there was no evidence of peripheral or entrapment neuropathy, and the deep tendon reflexes were normal. I asked Andrew to walk down the hall; there, I noted an antalgic gait was present.

Key Clinical Points—What's Important and What's Not

THE HISTORY

- Onset of left knee pain following laying carpeting
- Pain localized to the area of the left suprapatellar region
- Pain associated with swelling of the affected knee
- Pain made worse by squatting or kneeling on left
- No other specific traumatic event to the area identified
- History of mild self-limited left knee pain after kicking in carpeting
- No fever or chills

- Sleep disturbance
- Difficulty walking or squatting
- Unable to kneel on left knee

THE PHYSICAL EXAMINATION

- The patient is afebrile
- Point tenderness to palpation of the area over the suprapatellar bursa
- Palpation of left knee reveals warmth to touch
- The left lateral knee is swollen, with "bogginess"
- No evidence of infection
- Pain on range of motion, especially resisted extension and passive flexion of the affected left knee
- The resisted extension release test was positive on the left (see Fig. 7.1)
- An antalgic gait was present

OTHER FINDINGS OF NOTE

- Normal HEENT examination
- Normal cardiovascular examination
- Normal pulmonary examination
- Normal abdominal examination
- No tenderness to deep palpation of the lumbar paraspinous muscles
- No peripheral edema
- Normal upper and lower extremity neurologic examination, motor and sensory examination
- Examinations of joints other than the left knee were normal

What Tests Would You Like to Order?

The following tests were ordered:
- Plain radiographs of the left knee
- Ultrasound of the left knee

TEST RESULTS

The plain radiographs of the left knee revealed a fluid density behind the patellar tendon and around the patella tip, and patella tilting due to abundant effusion. No fracture or other bony abnormality was noted (Fig. 7.2). Ultrasound examination of the left knee revealed suprapatellar bursitis and plica formation. Osteophyte and patellofemoral degenerative changes are noted (Fig. 7.3).

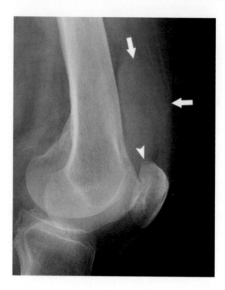

Fig. 7.2 Fluid density is present behind the patellar tendon and around patella tip *(arrows);* note patella tilting *(arrowhead)* due to abundant effusion. No fracture or other bony abnormality is noted. (From Venkatasamy A, Ehlinger M, Bierry G. Acute traumatic knee radiographs: beware of lesions of little expression but of great significance. *Diagn Interv Imaging.* 2014;95[6]:551–560, Fig. 3.)

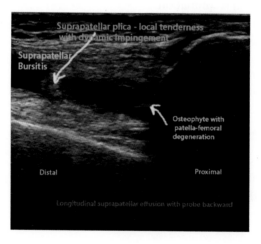

Fig. 7.3 Longitudinal ultrasound image demonstrating suprapatellar bursitis and plica formation. Note the osteophyte and patella-femoral degenerative changes. (From Waldman SD. *Atlas of Common Pain Syndromes.* 4th ed. Philadelphia: Elsevier; 2019: Fig. 112.3.)

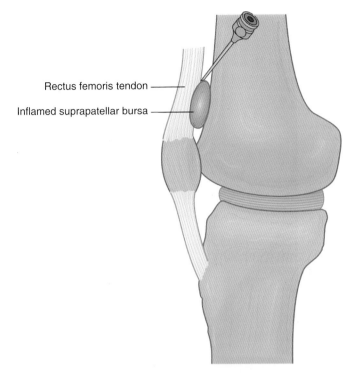

Rectus femoris tendon —————

Inflamed suprapatellar bursa —————

Fig. 7.4 The suprapatellar bursa lies between the anterior surface of the distal femur and the distal quadriceps musculotendinous unit. (From Waldman SD. *Atlas of Pain Management Injection Techniques*. 4th ed. St Louis: Elsevier; 2017: Fig. 140-2.)

Clinical Correlation—Putting It All Together

What is the diagnosis?
- Suprapatellar bursitis

The Science Behind the Diagnosis

ANATOMY

There is significant intrapatient variability in size of the suprapatellar bursa. The suprapatellar bursa lies between the anterior surface of the distal femur and the distal quadriceps musculotendinous unit (Fig. 7.4). The suprapatellar bursa is held in place by a small portion of the vastus intermedius muscle called the articularis genus muscle. Both the quadriceps tendon and the suprapatellar bursa are subject to the development of inflammation caused by overuse, misuse, or direct trauma (Fig. 7.5). The quadriceps tendon is made up of fibers from the four muscles that

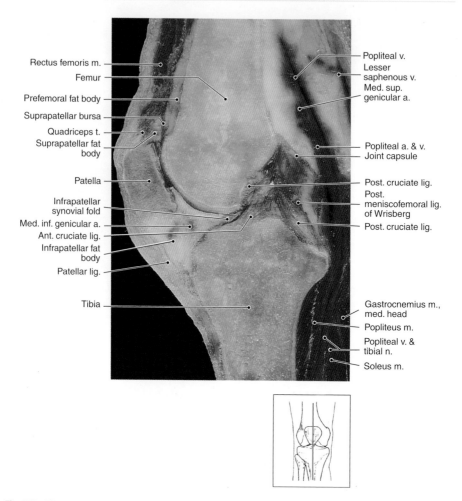

Rectus femoris m.
Femur
Prefemoral fat body
Suprapatellar bursa
Quadriceps t.
Suprapatellar fat body
Patella
Infrapatellar synovial fold
Med. inf. genicular a.
Ant. cruciate lig.
Infrapatellar fat body
Patellar lig.
Tibia

Popliteal v.
Lesser saphenous v.
Med. sup. genicular a.
Popliteal a. & v.
Joint capsule
Post. cruciate lig.
Post. meniscofemoral lig. of Wrisberg
Post. cruciate lig.
Gastrocnemius m., med. head
Popliteus m.
Popliteal v. & tibial n.
Soleus m.

Fig. 7.5   The suprapatellar bursa serves to cushion and facilitate sliding of the musculotendinous unit of the quadriceps muscle over the distal femur. (From Waldman SD. *Atlas of Pain Management Injection Techniques*. 4th ed. St Louis: Elsevier; 2017: Fig. 140-1.)

comprise the quadriceps muscle: the vastus lateralis, the vastus intermedius, the vastus medialis, and the rectus femoris. These muscles are the primary extensors of the lower extremity at the knee. The tendons of these muscles converge and unite to form a single, exceedingly strong tendon. The patella functions as a sesamoid bone within the quadriceps tendon, with fibers of the tendon expanding around the patella and forming the medial and lateral patella retinacula, which help strengthen the knee joint. These fibers are called expansions and are subject to strain; the tendon proper is subject to the development of tendinitis. The suprapatellar, infrapatellar, and prepatellar bursae also may concurrently become inflamed with dysfunction of the quadriceps and patellar tendon.

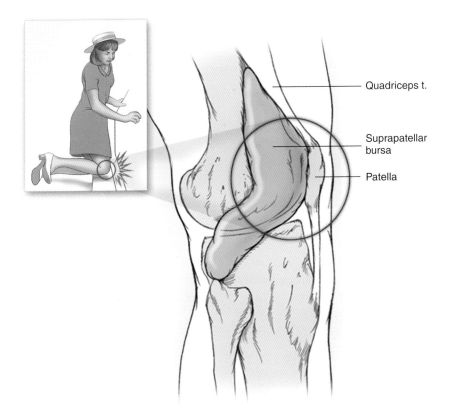

Quadriceps t.

Suprapatellar bursa

Patella

Fig. 7.6 Suprapatellar bursitis is usually the result of direct trauma from either acute injury or repeated microtrauma, such as prolonged kneeling. (From Waldman SD. *Atlas of Common Pain Syndromes.* 4th ed. Philadelphia: Elsevier; 2019: Fig. 112-1.)

CLINICAL SYNDROME

Suprapatellar bursitis is a common cause of anterior knee pain. The suprapatellar bursa lies between the anterior surface of the distal femur and the distal quadriceps musculotendinous unit (see Fig. 7.4). The bursa serves to cushion and facilitate sliding of the musculotendinous unit of the quadriceps muscle over the distal femur. The bursa is subject to inflammation from a variety of causes, with acute trauma to the knee and repetitive microtrauma being the most common. Acute injuries to the bursa can occur from direct blunt trauma to the anterior knee from falls onto the knee as well as from overuse injuries, including running on uneven or soft surfaces or jobs that require kneeling or crawling on the knees, such as laying carpet (Fig. 7.6). If the inflammation of the bursa is not treated and the condition becomes chronic, calcification of the bursa with further functional

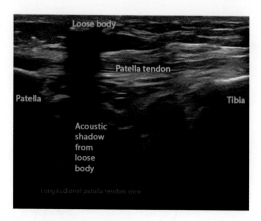

Loose body

Patella tendon

Patella

Tibia

Acoustic
shadow
from
loose
body

Longitudinal patella tendon view

Fig. 7.7 Longitudinal tendon ultrasound image demonstrating a joint mouse.

disability may occur. Gout and other crystal arthropathies may also precipitate acute suprapatellar bursitis, as may loose bodies and bacterial, tubercular, or fungal infections (Fig. 7.7).

SIGNS AND SYMPTOMS

The patient suffering from suprapatellar bursitis most frequently presents with the complaint of pain in the anterior knee, which may radiate superiorly into the distal thigh. The patient may find walking down stairs and kneeling increasingly difficult. Physical examination of the patient suffering from suprapatellar bursitis will reveal point tenderness over the superior anterior knee. If there is significant inflammation, rubor and color may be present, and the entire area may feel boggy or edematous to palpation. Active resisted extension and passive flexion of the affected knee will often reproduce the patient's pain (see Fig. 7.1). Sudden release of resistance to active extension will markedly increase the pain. If calcification or gouty tophi of the bursa and surrounding tendons is present, the examiner may appreciate crepitus with active extension of the knee, and the patient may complain of a catching sensation when moving the affected knee, especially on awakening. Often, the patient will not be able to sleep on the affected side. Occasionally, the suprapatellar bursa may become infected, with systemic symptoms, including fever and malaise, as well as local symptoms, with rubor, color, and dolor being present.

TESTING

Plain radiographs are indicated in all patients who present with knee pain to rule out occult bony pathology (see Fig. 7.2). Based on the patient's clinical presentation, additional testing may be indicated, including complete blood cell

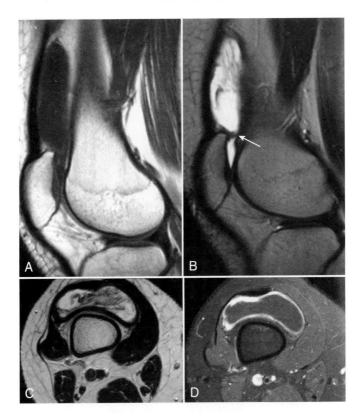

Fig. 7.8 Sagittal T1 weighted (T1W) (A) and T2W (B) magnetic resonance (MR) images of a patient with an imperforate superior plica *(white arrow)*. There is a loculated effusion within the suprapatellar bursa but no significant effusion in the other recesses of the knee joint. A few low signal intensity (SI) fronds of synovium within the bursa can be seen on the sagittal T2W MR image and on an axial T2W MR image (C). (D) An axial T1W with fat suppression (FST1W) MR image obtained after administration of a contrast agent shows minor enhancement of the synovial lining of the bursa. (From Waldman SD, Campbell RSD. *Imaging of Pain*. Philadelphia: Saunders; 2011: Fig. 156.1.)

count, sedimentation rate, and antinuclear antibody testing. Magnetic resonance imaging (MRI) or ultrasound imaging of the affected area may also confirm the diagnosis and help delineate the presence of other knee bursitis, calcific tendinitis, tendinopathy, triceps tendinitis, or other knee pathology (Figs. 7.8, 7.9, and 7.10). Rarely, the inflamed bursa may become infected, and failure to diagnose and treat the acute infection can lead to dire consequences (Fig. 7.11).

DIFFERENTIAL DIAGNOSIS

Because of the anatomy of the region, the associated tendons and other bursae of the knee can become inflamed along with the suprapatellar bursa, thus

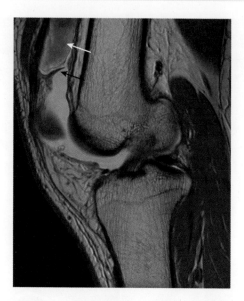

Fig. 7.9 Sagittal T2 weighted (T2W) magnetic resonance (MR) image of an imperforate plica *(black arrow)* in a patient with a loculated hematoma in the suprapatellar bursa *(white arrow)* following an acute injury. (From Waldman SD, Campbell RSD. *Imaging of Pain*. Philadelphia: Saunders; 2011: Fig. 156.2.)

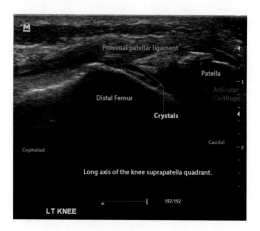

Fig. 7.10 Ultrasound image demonstrating crystal deposition disease of the knee.

confusing the diagnosis. Both the quadriceps tendon and the suprapatellar bursa are subject to inflammation from overuse, misuse, or direct trauma. The tendon fibers, called expansions, are vulnerable to strain, and the tendon proper is subject to the development of tendinitis. The suprapatellar, infrapatellar, and prepatellar bursae may also become inflamed with dysfunction of the quadriceps

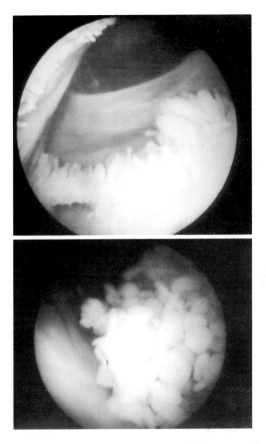

Fig. 7.11 Arthroscopic views of rice bodies within the intraarticular space of a septic knee. (From Aşik M, Eralp L, Çetik O, et al. Rice bodies of synovial origin in the knee joint. *Arthroscopy J Arthroscopic Related Surgery*. 2001;17[5]:1—4, Fig. 2.)

tendon. Anything that alters the normal biomechanics of the knee can result in inflammation of the suprapatellar bursa (Table 7.1).

TREATMENT

A short course of conservative therapy consisting of simple analgesics, nonsteroidal antiinflammatory drugs (NSAIDs), or cyclooxygenase-2 inhibitors and a knee brace to prevent further trauma is the first step in the treatment of suprapatellar bursitis. If patients do not experience rapid improvement, injection is a reasonable next step.

To perform the injection, the patient is placed in the supine position with a rolled blanket underneath the knee to flex the joint gently. The skin overlying the

---

TABLE 7.1 ■ **Differential Diagnosis of Suprapatellar Bursitis**

- Arthritides of the knee
- Patellar abnormalities
- Tendinopathies
- Ligamentous strain
- Avascular necrosis of the knee joint
- Septic arthritis
- Impingement syndromes
- Fractures of the tibial plateau
- Avulsion fractures around the knee
- Iliotibial band inflammation
- Osgood-Schlatter disease
- Complex regional pain syndrome

---

medial aspect of the knee joint is prepared with antiseptic solution. A sterile syringe containing 2 mL of 0.25% preservative-free bupivacaine and 40 mg methylprednisolone is attached to a 1.5-inch, 25-gauge needle using strict aseptic technique. The superior margin of the medial patella is identified. Just above this point, the needle is inserted horizontally to slide beneath the quadriceps tendon. If the needle strikes the femur, it is withdrawn slightly and is redirected with a more anterior trajectory. When the needle is in position just below the quadriceps tendon, the contents of the syringe are gently injected (see Fig. 7.4). Little resistance to injection should be felt. If resistance is encountered, the needle is probably in a ligament or tendon and should be advanced or withdrawn slightly until the injection can proceed without significant resistance. The needle is removed, and a sterile pressure dressing and ice pack are applied to the injection site. Ultrasound needle guidance will improve the accuracy of needle placement and decrease the incidence of needle-induced complications.

Physical modalities, including local heat and gentle range of motion exercises, should be introduced several days after the patient undergoes injection. Vigorous exercises should be avoided because they will exacerbate the patient's symptoms. Simple analgesics and NSAIDs can be used concurrently with this injection technique.

HIGH-YIELD TAKEAWAYS

- The patient is afebrile, making an acute infectious etiology (e.g., septic arthritis) unlikely.
- The patient's symptomatology is the result of acute trauma. Physical examination and testing should be focused on the identification of ligamentous injury, acute arthritis, tendinitis, and bursitis.

(Continued)

- The patient has point tenderness over the suprapatellar bursa, which is highly suggestive of suprapatellar bursitis.
- There is warmth and swelling of the area overlying the suprapatellar bursa, suggestive of an inflammatory process.
- The patient's symptoms are unilateral and involve only one joint, which is more suggestive of a local process than a systemic polyarthropathy.
- Sleep disturbance is common and must be addressed concurrently with the patient's pain symptomatology.
- Plain radiographs will provide high-yield information regarding the bony contents of the joint and the identification of fractures or other bony abnormalities of the femur as well as calcification of the bursa and tendons, but ultrasound imaging and MRI will be more useful in identifying soft tissue pathology.

Suggested Readings

Waldman SD. Bursitis syndromes of the knee. In: *Pain Review*. 2nd ed. Philadelphia: Elsevier; 2017:306–308.

Waldman SD. Injection technique for suprapatellar bursitis. In: *Pain Review*. Philadelphia: Saunders; 2009:584–585.

Waldman SD. Injection technique for suprapatellar bursitis. In: *Pain Review*. 2nd ed. Philadelphia: Elsevier; 2017. 717–716.

Waldman SD. Suprapatellar bursitis. In: *Waldman's Comprehensive Atlas of Diagnostic Ultrasound of Painful Conditions*. 1st ed. Philadelphia: Wolters Kluwer; 2016:780–785.

Waldman SD. Suprapatellar bursitis and other disorders of the suprapatellar bursa. In: *Waldman's Comprehensive Atlas of Diagnostic Ultrasound of Painful Conditions*. 1st ed. Philadelphia: Wolters Kluwer; 2016:206–217.

Waldman SD. Suprapatellar bursa injection. 4th ed. In: *Atlas of Pain Management Injection Techniques*. 417-419. Philadelphia: Elsevier; 2017:523–526.

Waldman SD. The suprapatellar bursa. In: *Pain Review*. 2nd ed. Philadelphia: Elsevier; 2017:303–304.

Waldman SD. Ultrasound-guided injection technique for suprapatellar bursitis. In: *Comprehensive Atlas of Ultrasound Guided Pain Management Injection Techniques*. 1st ed. Philadelphia: Lippincott; 2014:810–816.

Waldman SD, Campbell RSD. Anatomy: special imaging considerations of the knee. In: *Imaging of Pain*. Philadelphia: Saunders; 2011:367–388.

Waldman SD, Campbell RSD. Anatomy: suprapatellar bursitis. In: *Imaging of Pain*. 1st ed. Philadelphia: Saunders; 2011:401–402.

Betsy Roos

A 27-Year-Old Homemaker With Severe Left Knee Pain and Swelling

- Learn the common causes of knee pain.
- Develop an understanding of the unique anatomy of the knee joint.
- Develop an understanding of the bursae of the knee.
- Develop an understanding of the causes of prepatellar bursitis.
- Develop an understanding of the differential diagnosis of prepatellar bursitis.
- Learn the clinical presentation of prepatellar bursitis.
- Learn how to examine the knee and associated bursae.
- Learn how to use physical examination to identify prepatellar bursitis.
- Develop an understanding of the treatment options for prepatellar bursitis.

Betsy Roos

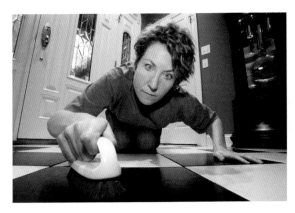

Betsy Roos is a 27-year-old homemaker with the chief complaint of, "My left knee is bigger than my head." Betsy stated that over the past several weeks, her left knee started "swelling up like a balloon." She went on to say, "It is all my mother-in-law's fault." I said, "So how is your swollen knee your mother-in-law's fault"? Betsy laughed and said that her mother-in-law was coming for a visit and she had been scrubbing the house from top to bottom. "Doc, have you ever got down on your hands and knees and used a toothbrush to scrub around the toilets, the baseboards, the corners? I bet you haven't, and if you do, then your knee will be bigger than your head, too!" I laughed and asked her if she ever had anything like this before and she said, "The mother-in-law or the knee?" I laughed again and said, "The knee, Betsy, the knee." She just shook her head and said, "No, never, and I don't want it ever again. It really hurts and it is really hard to walk down the stairs to the basement to throw in a load of laundry. I sure as hell am not letting my husband anywhere near the washing machine. The last time he did laundry, he threw in a brand new red t-shirt with my delicates and now I have a collection of amazing pink unmentionables, so no way. Doc, my knee is so swollen I can't really see my kneecap anymore. That is really not the look I am going for!"

I asked Betsy what made the pain worse and she said any walking, stairs (going down was worse than going up, but going up still hurt), putting on socks, squatting, and "getting down on my left knee is completely out of the question." I asked her what made it better and she said Advil seemed to help, but it was upsetting her stomach. She noted that the heating pad felt good, but she thought it made her knee swell more. I asked Betsy about any antecedent knee trauma and she said, "Nothing I can remember." Betsy volunteered that trying to get to sleep was "a real pain in the keister" because every time she moved her left leg, her knee would really hurt.

I asked Betsy to point with one finger to show me where it hurt the most. She pointed to one of the most swollen knees I had ever seen (she really wasn't kidding when she said the knee was as big as her head—it literally was no exaggeration) (Fig. 8.1).

On physical examination, Betsy was afebrile. Her respirations were 16 and her pulse was 74 and regular. Her blood pressure was 126/76. Betsy's head,

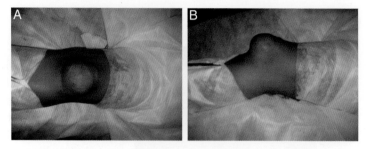

Fig. 8.1 Prepatellar bursitis. (A) Clinical photograph of a patient with prepatellar bursitis as viewed from the anterior aspect and (B) as viewed from the side. (From Arora S, Batra S, Rao S, Maini L, Gautam VK. A 40-year-old female with painless, slow growing prepatellar mass. *J Clin Orthop Trauma.* 2014;5(4):274–279.)

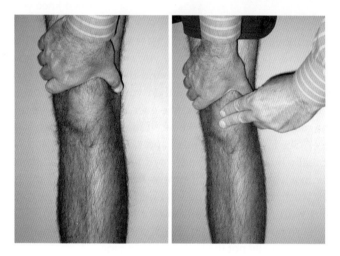

Fig. 8.2 The ballottement test for large joint effusions. (From Waldman SD. *Physical Diagnosis of Pain: An Atlas of Signs and Symptoms.* 3rd ed. St Louis: Elsevier; 2016: 203-1.)

eyes, ears, nose, and throat (HEENT) exam was normal, as was her cardiopulmonary examination. Her thyroid was normal. Her abdominal examination revealed no abnormal mass or organomegaly. There was no costovertebral angle (CVA) tenderness. There was no peripheral edema. Her low back examination revealed some tenderness to deep palpation of the paraspinous musculature. Visual inspection of the left knee revealed massive swelling. The area over the left prepatellar area felt warm but did not appear to be infected. The left knee felt "boggy" on palpation. There was a positive ballottement test on the left (Fig. 8.2). There was marked tenderness to palpation over the prepatellar region, with palpation of the area exacerbating Betsy's pain. Range of motion of the knee joint, especially resisted extension and passive flexion of the knee joint, caused Betsy to cry out in pain. The right knee examination was normal, as was examination of her major joints. A careful neurologic examination of the upper and lower extremities revealed there was no evidence of peripheral or entrapment neuropathy, and the deep tendon reflexes were normal. I asked Betsy to walk down the hall, and there, I noted an antalgic gait was present.

Key Clinical Points—What's Important and What's Not

THE HISTORY

- Onset of left knee pain following scrubbing floors on her hands and knees
- Pain localized to the area of the left prepatellar region
- Pain associated with swelling of the affected knee
- Pain made worse by squatting or kneeling on left
- No other specific traumatic event to the area identified
- No fever or chills
- Sleep disturbance
- Difficulty walking and squatting
- Unable to kneel on left knee

THE PHYSICAL EXAMINATION

- The patient is afebrile
- Point tenderness to palpation of the area over the prepatellar bursa
- Palpation of left knee reveals warmth to touch
- The left knee is swollen, with "bogginess"
- No evidence of infection
- Pain on range of motion, especially resisted extension and passive flexion of the affected left knee
- The ballottement test was positive on the left (see Fig. 8.2)
- An antalgic gait was present

OHER FINDINGS OF NOTE

- Normal HEENT examination
- Normal cardiovascular examination
- Normal pulmonary examination
- Normal abdominal examination
- No tenderness to deep palpation of the lumbar paraspinous muscles
- No peripheral edema
- Normal upper and lower extremity neurologic examination, motor and sensory examination
- Examination of joints other than the left knee were normal

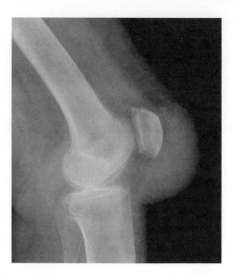

Fig. 8.3 Lateral radiograph reveals a large prepatellar fluid collection. (From Waldman SD, Campbell RSD. *Imaging of Pain*. Philadelphia: Elsevier; 2011.)

 ## What Tests Would You Like to Order?

The following tests were ordered:
- Plain radiographs of the left knee
- Ultrasound of the left knee

TEST RESULTS

The plain radiographs of the left knee reveal a large prepatellar fluid collection (Fig. 8.3). Ultrasound examination of the left knee revealed prepatellar bursitis and plica formation. Osteophyte and patellofemoral degenerative changes are noted (Fig. 8.4).

Clinical Correlation—Putting It All Together

What is the diagnosis?
- Prepatellar bursitis

The Science Behind the Diagnosis
ANATOMY

The prepatellar bursa lies between the subcutaneous tissues and the patella (Fig. 8.5). The bursa is held in place by the ligamentum patellae. Both the

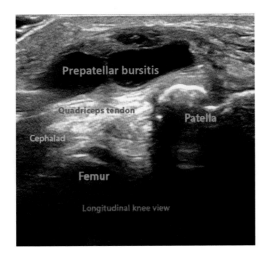

Fig 8.4 Longitudinal ultrasound image demonstrating a large prepatellar bursitis. (From Waldman SD. *Atlas of Common Pain Syndromes*. 4th ed. Philadelphia: Elsevier; 2019: Fig. 113.7.)

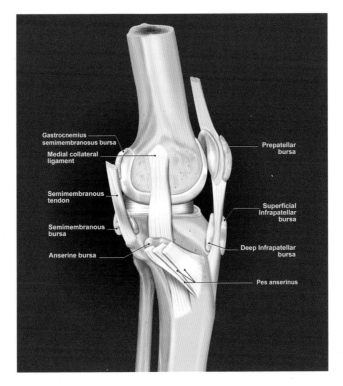

Fig. 8.5 The prepatellar bursa lies between the subcutaneous tissues and the patella. (From Lormeau C, Cormier G, Sigaux J, et al. Management of septic bursitis. *Joint Bone Spine*. 2019;86[5]:583–588, Fig. 1.)

quadriceps tendon and the prepatellar bursa are subject to the development of inflammation following overuse, misuse, or direct trauma. The quadriceps tendon is made up of fibers from the four muscles that comprise the quadriceps muscle: the vastus lateralis, the vastus intermedius, the vastus medialis, and the rectus femoris. These muscles are the primary extensors of the lower extremity at the knee. The tendons of these muscles converge and unite to form a single, exceedingly strong tendon (Fig. 8.6). The patella functions as a sesamoid bone within the quadriceps tendon with fibers of the tendon expanding around the patella forming the medial and lateral patellar retinacula, which help strengthen the knee joint. These fibers are called expansions and are subject to strain, and the tendon proper is subject to the development of tendinitis. The suprapatellar, infrapatellar, and prepatellar bursa may also concurrently become inflamed with dysfunction of the quadriceps tendon.

CLINICAL SYNDROME

The prepatellar bursa lies between the subcutaneous tissues and the patella. This bursa is held in place by the patellar ligament. The prepatellar bursa may exist as a single bursal sac or, in some patients, as a multisegmented series of loculated sacs (Fig. 8.7). The prepatellar bursa is vulnerable to injury from both acute trauma and repeated microtrauma. Acute injuries are caused by direct trauma to the bursa during falls onto the knee or patellar fracture. Overuse injuries may be caused by running on soft or uneven surfaces or jobs that require crawling or kneeling, such as laying carpet or scrubbing floors, hence the other name for prepatellar bursitis: housemaid's knee (Fig. 8.8). If inflammation of the prepatellar bursa becomes chronic, calcification may occur.

SIGNS AND SYMPTOMS

Patients suffering from prepatellar bursitis complain of pain and swelling in the anterior knee over the patella that can radiate superiorly and inferiorly into the surrounding area (Fig. 8.9; see Fig. 8.1). Often, patients are unable to kneel or walk down stairs. Patients may also complain of a sharp "catching" sensation with range of motion of the knee, especially on first arising. Prepatellar bursitis often coexists with arthritis and tendinitis of the knee, which can confuse the clinical picture.

TESTING

Plain radiographs and magnetic resonance imaging (MRI) of the knee may reveal calcification of the bursa and associated structures, including the

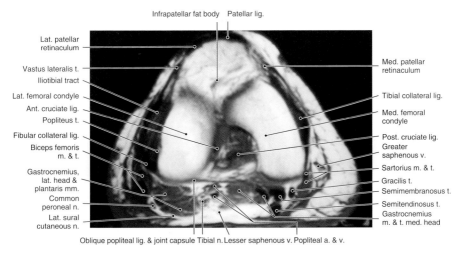

Infrapatellar fat body   Patellar lig.

Lat. patellar retinaculum

Vastus lateralis t.
Iliotibial tract
Lat. femoral condyle
Ant. cruciate lig.
Popliteus t.
Fibular collateral lig.
Biceps femoris m. & t.
Gastrocnemius, lat. head & plantaris mm.
Common peroneal n.
Lat. sural cutaneous n.

Med. patellar retinaculum

Tibial collateral lig.
Med. femoral condyle
Post. cruciate lig.
Greater saphenous v.
Sartorius m. & t.
Gracilis t.
Semimembranosus t.
Semitendinosus t.
Gastrocnemius m. & t. med. head

Oblique popliteal lig. & joint capsule Tibial n. Lesser saphenous v. Popliteal a. & v.

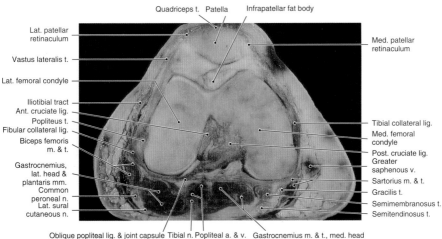

Quadriceps t.   Patella   Infrapatellar fat body

Lat. patellar retinaculum

Vastus lateralis t.

Lat. femoral condyle

Iliotibial tract
Ant. cruciate lig.
Popliteus t.
Fibular collateral lig.
Biceps femoris m. & t.
Gastrocnemius, lat. head & plantaris mm.
Common peroneal n.
Lat. sural cutaneous n.

Med. patellar retinaculum

Tibial collateral lig.
Med. femoral condyle
Post. cruciate lig.
Greater saphenous v.
Sartorius m. & t.
Gracilis t.
Semimembranosus t.
Semitendinosus t.

Oblique popliteal lig. & joint capsule Tibial n. Popliteal a. & v. Gastrocnemius m. & t., med. head

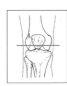

Fig. 8.6 Anatomy of the quadriceps tendon and related structures. *ant.*, Anterior; *lat.*, lateral; *lig.*, ligament; *m./mm*, muscle/muscles; *med.*, medial; *n.*, nerve; *post.*, posterior; *t.*, tendon; *v.*, vein. (From Kang HS, Ahn JM, Resnick D. *MRI of the Extremities: An Anatomic Atlas*. 2nd edition. Philadelphia: Saunders; 2002.)

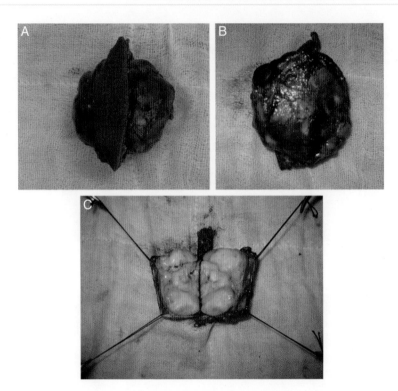

Fig. 8.7 (A) Resected specimen of prepatellar bursitis (size: 5.5 cm × 4 cm × 5 cm) with overlying redundant skin, pseudocapsule, and a margin of healthy tissue. (B) The posterior surface of the specimen along with pseudocapsule and periosteum of patella and sheath of patellar tendon. (C) The cut surface of the mass (cut open from the posterior surface) showing a well-circumscribed, trilobulated, yellowish-white fibrous structure without macroscopic areas of hemorrhage or necrosis. (From Arora S, Batra S, Rao S, Maini L, Gautam VK. A 40-year-old female with painless, slow growing prepatellar mass. *J Clin Orthop Trauma*. 2014;5(4):274–279.)

quadriceps tendon, consistent with chronic inflammation (see Fig. 8.3). They may also reveal evidence of infection (Fig. 8.10). MRI and ultrasound imaging is indicated if internal derangement, an occult mass, infection, or a tumor of the knee is suspected, and to help clarify the diagnosis (Figs. 8.11, 8.12, and 8.13). Electromyography can distinguish prepatellar bursitis from femoral neuropathy, lumbar radiculopathy, and plexopathy. The injection technique described later serves as both a diagnostic and a therapeutic maneuver. Antinuclear antibody testing is indicated if collagen vascular disease is suspected. If infection is a possibility, aspiration, Gram stain, and culture of bursal fluid should be performed on an emergency basis.

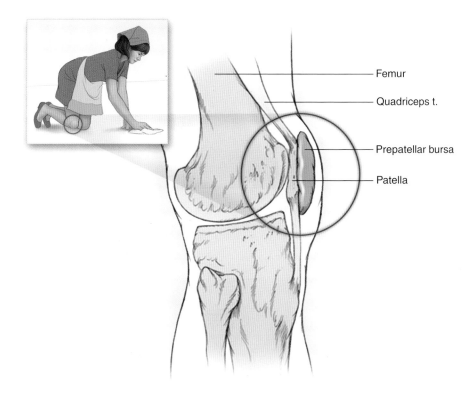

Femur

Quadriceps t.

Prepatellar bursa

Patella

Fig. 8.8 Prepatellar bursitis is also known as housemaid's knee because of its prevalence among people whose work requires prolonged crawling or kneeling. (From Waldman SD. *Atlas of Common Pain Syndromes*. 4th ed. Philadelphia: Elsevier; 2019: Fig. 113.2.)

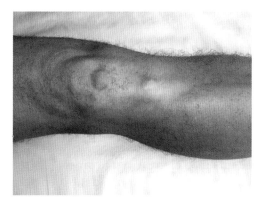

Fig. 8.9 Mild prepatellar bursitis. (Courtesy Steven Waldman, MD.)

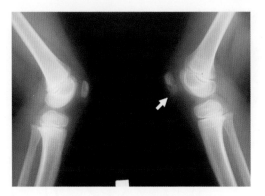

Fig. 8.10   Radiograph of the knee in a patient suspected of having septic prepatellar bursitis depicts fragmentation and elongation of the patella, consistent with osteomyelitis of the patella *(arrow)*. (From Choi H-R. Patellar osteomyelitis presenting as prepatellar bursitis. *Knee*. 2007;14[4]:333−335, Fig. 5.)

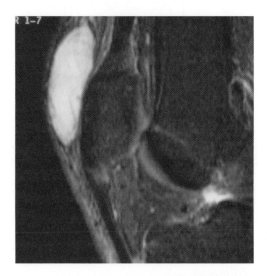

Fig. 8.11   Prepatellar bursitis. A sagittal short tau inversion recovery (TR/TE, 5300/30; inversion time, 150 ms) magnetic resonance image shows fluid and synovial tissue in the prepatellar bursa. (From Resnick D. *Diagnosis of Bone and Joint Disorders*. 4th ed. Philadelphia: Saunders; 2002.)

DIFFERENTIAL DIAGNOSIS

Because of the anatomy of the region, the associated tendons and other bursae of the knee can become inflamed along with the prepatellar bursa, thus confusing the diagnosis. Both the quadriceps tendon and the prepatellar bursa are subject to inflammation from overuse, misuse, or direct trauma. The tendon fibers, called expansions, are vulnerable to strain, and the tendon proper is subject to the development of tendinitis. The suprapatellar, infrapatellar, and prepatellar bursae may also become inflamed with dysfunction of the quadriceps tendon.

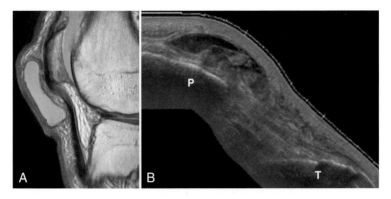

Fig. 8.12 Magentic resonance (MR) image of prepatellar bursitis coexistent with patellofemoral osteoarthritis. (A) Sagittal T2 weighted (T2W) MR image showing prominent high signal intensity (SI) fluid within the prepatellar bursa. Here is also an advanced osteoarthritic change in the patellofemoral joint. (B) The corresponding longitudinal ultrasound image shows the extensive low-echo fluid collection. *P*, Patella; *T*, tibia. (From Waldman SD, Campbell RSD. *Imaging of Pain*. Philadelphia: Elsevier; 2011.)

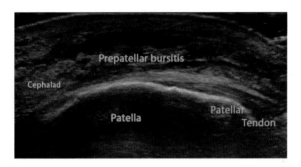

Fig. 8.13 Longitudinal ultrasound image demonstrating prepatellar bursitis. (Courtesy Steven Waldman, MD.)

Anything that alters the normal biomechanics of the knee can result in inflammation of the prepatellar bursa.

TREATMENT

A short course of conservative therapy consisting of simple analgesics, nonsteroidal antiinflammatory drugs, or cyclooxygenase-2 inhibitors and a knee brace to prevent further trauma is the first step in the treatment of prepatellar bursitis. If patients do not experience rapid improvement, injection of local anesthetic and steroid is a reasonable next step. Ultrasound needle guidance will improve the accuracy of needle placement and decrease the incidence of needle-related complications.

HIGH-YIELD TAKEAWAYS

- The patient is afebrile, making an acute infectious etiology (e.g., septic arthritis) unlikely.
- The patient's symptomatology is the result of acute trauma and physical examination, and testing should be focused on the identification of ligamentous injury, acute arthritis, tendinitis, and bursitis.
- The patient has point tenderness over the prepatellar bursa, which is highly suggestive of prepatellar bursitis.
- There is warmth and swelling of the area overlying the prepatellar bursa, suggestive of an inflammatory process.
- The patient's symptoms are unilateral and involve only one joint, which is more suggestive of a local process than a systemic polyarthropathy.
- Sleep disturbance is common and must be addressed concurrently with the patient's pain symptomatology.
- Plain radiographs will provide high-yield information regarding the bony contents of the joint and the identification of fractures or other bony abnormalities of the femur as well as calcification of the bursa and tendons, but ultrasound imaging and MRI will be more useful in identifying soft tissue pathology.

Suggested Readings

Steinbach LS, Stevens KJ. Imaging of cysts and bursae about the knee. *Radiol Clin N Am*. 2013;51(3):433–454.

Waldman SD. Bursitis syndromes of the knee. In: *Pain Review*. 2nd ed. Philadelphia: Elsevier; 2017:306–308.

Waldman SD. Prepatellar bursa injection. In: *Atlas of Pain Management Injection Techniques*. 4th ed. Philadelphia, PA: Elsevier; 2017:449–452.

Waldman SD. Prepatellar bursitis. In: *Waldman's Comprehensive Atlas of Diagnostic Ultrasound of Painful Conditions*. 1st ed. Philadelphia: Wolters Kluwer; 2016:786–791.

Waldman SD. Prepatellar bursitis and other disorders of the prepatellar bursa. In: *Waldman's Comprehensive Atlas of Diagnostic Ultrasound of Painful Conditions*. 1st ed. Philadelphia: Wolters Kluwer; 2016:218–224.

Waldman SD, Campbell RSD. Anatomy: special imaging considerations of the knee. In: *Imaging of Pain*. 1st ed. Philadelphia: Saunders; 2011:367–388.

Waldman SD, Campbell RSD. Prepatellar bursitis. In: *Imaging of Pain*. 1st ed. Philadelphia: Saunders; 2011:405–406.

Arif Abad

A 29-Year-Old Electrical Engineer With Severe Left Knee and Upper Leg Pain and Swelling

LEARNING OBJECTIVES

- Learn the common causes of knee pain.
- Develop an understanding of the unique anatomy of the knee joint.
- Develop an understanding of the bursae of the knee.
- Develop an understanding of the causes of deep infrapatellar bursitis.
- Develop an understanding of the differential diagnosis of deep infrapatellar bursitis.
- Learn the clinical presentation of deep infrapatellar bursitis.
- Learn how to examine the knee and associated bursae.
- Learn how to use physical examination to identify deep infrapatellar bursitis.
- Develop an understanding of the treatment options for deep infrapatellar bursitis.

Arif Abad

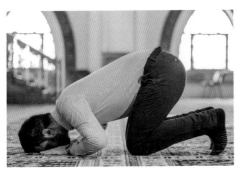

Arif Abad is a 29-year-old electrical engineer with the chief complaint of, "My left knee is really bothering me." Arif stated that over the last few weeks, he began having left knee pain and swelling. "I don't know whether I injured my knee when I was exercising or I just slept on it wrong. I really notice the pain when I do my morning prayers. I tried to take it easy with the jogging and have been taking Motrin around the clock, but when I kneel during my prayers, it really hurts. By the time I get home from work, my knee is really swollen. The heating pad helps a bit, but the swelling really concerns me."

I asked Arif about any antecedent knee trauma and he just shook his head no. "I really try to watch what I eat and be sure that my running shoes are in good shape to protect my joints." "Good to hear, Arif. What kinds of things make your pain and swelling worse?" I asked. "Doctor, any time I put weight on my knee, try to run, or pray, I really feel it."

I asked Arif to point with one finger to show me where it hurt the most. He pointed to the area just below the left patella and said, "Doctor, it's right here!"

On physical examination, Arif was afebrile. His respirations were 18 and his pulse was 96 and regular. His blood pressure was 138/98. Arif's head, eyes, ears, nose, and throat (HEENT) exam was normal, as was his cardiopulmonary examination. His thyroid was normal. His abdominal examination revealed no abnormal mass or organomegaly. There was no costovertebral angle (CVA) tenderness. There was no peripheral edema. His low back examination revealed some tenderness to deep palpation of the paraspinous musculature. Visual inspection of the left lateral knee revealed moderate swelling. The area over the left deep infrapatellar area felt a little warm but did not appear to be infected. The left knee felt "boggy" on palpation, and there was marked tenderness to palpation over the deep infrapatellar region. Palpation of this area exacerbated Arif's pain. Range of motion of the knee joint, especially with resisted extension and passive flexion of the knee joint, caused Arif to cry out in pain. I performed the active resisted extension release test, which was markedly positive on the left and negative on the right (Fig. 9.1). The right knee examination was normal, as was examination of Arif's major joints. A careful neurologic examination of the upper and lower extremities revealed there was no evidence of peripheral or

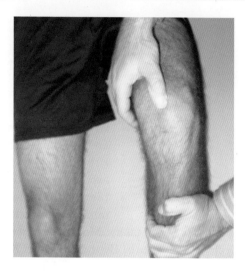

Fig. 9.1 The active resisted extension release test for deep infrapatellar bursitis. (From Waldman SD. *Physical Diagnosis of Pain: An Atlas of Signs and Symptoms*. 3rd ed. St Louis: Elsevier; 2016: Fig. 224-3.)

entrapment neuropathy, and the deep tendon reflexes were normal. I asked Arif to walk down the hall, where I noted an antalgic gait was present.

Key Clinical Points—What's Important and What's Not

THE HISTORY

- Onset of left knee pain following praying
- Pain localized to the area of the left deep infrapatellar region
- Pain associated with swelling of the affected knee
- Pain made worse by squatting or kneeling on left
- No other specific traumatic event to the area identified
- History of mild, self-limited left knee pain after praying
- No fever or chills
- Sleep disturbance
- Difficulty walking or squatting
- Unable to kneel on left knee

THE PHYSICAL EXAMINATION

- The patient is afebrile
- Point tenderness to palpation of the area over the deep infrapatellar bursa
- Palpation of left knee reveals warmth to touch

- The left lateral knee is swollen, with "bogginess"
- No evidence of infection
- Pain on range of motion, especially resisted extension and passive flexion of the affected left knee
- The active resisted extension release test was positive on the left (see Fig. 9.1)
- An antalgic gait was present

OTHER FINDINGS OF NOTE

- Normal HEENT examination
- Normal cardiovascular examination
- Normal pulmonary examination
- Normal abdominal examination
- No tenderness to deep palpation of the lumbar paraspinous muscles
- No peripheral edema
- Normal upper and lower extremity neurologic examination, motor and sensory examination
- Examinations of joints other than the left knee were normal

 What Tests Would You Like to Order?

The following tests were ordered:
- Plain radiographs of the left knee
- Ultrasound of the left knee

TEST RESULTS

The plain radiographs of the left knee revealed no fracture or bony abnormality. Ultrasound examination of the left knee revealed deep infrapatellar bursitis (Fig. 9.2).

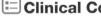 Clinical Correlation—Putting It All Together

What is the diagnosis?
- Deep infrapatellar bursitis

The Science Behind the Diagnosis

ANATOMY

There is significant intrapatient variability in size of the deep infrapatellar bursa. The deep infrapatellar bursa lies between the anterior subcutaneous tissues of

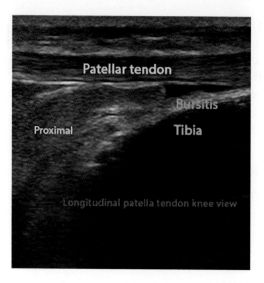

Fig. 9.2   Longitudinal ultrasound image demonstrating deep infrapatellar bursitis. (Courtesy Steven Waldman, MD.)

the knee and the anterior surface of the patellar tendon (Fig. 9.3). The bursa serves to cushion and facilitate sliding of the skin and subcutaneous tissues of the anterior inferior portion of the knee over the tibia. The deep infrapatellar bursa is held in place by patellar tendon, which is an extension of the common tendon of the quadriceps tendon. Both the quadriceps tendon and its expansions and the patellar tendon and the deep infrapatellar bursa are subject to the development of inflammation caused by overuse, misuse, or direct trauma. The quadriceps tendon is made up of fibers from the four muscles that comprise the quadriceps muscle: the vastus lateralis, the vastus intermedius, the vastus medialis, and the rectus femoris (Fig. 9.4). These muscles are the primary extensors of the lower extremity at the knee. The tendons of these muscles converge and unite to form a single, exceedingly strong tendon. The patella functions as a sesamoid bone within the quadriceps tendon, with fibers of the tendon expanding around the patella and forming the medial and lateral patella retinacula, which help strengthen the knee joint. These fibers are called expansions and are subject to strain; the tendon proper is subject to the development of tendonitis. The deep infrapatellar, deep infrapatellar, and prepatellar bursae also may concurrently become inflamed with dysfunction of the quadriceps tendon dysfunction.

CLINICAL SYNDROME

The deep infrapatellar bursa lies between the patellar ligament and the tibia. This bursa may exist as a single bursal sac or, in some patients, as a multisegmented

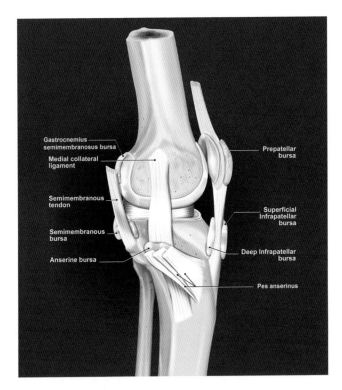

Fig. 9.3   The deep infrapatellar bursa lies between the anterior subcutaneous tissues of the knee and the anterior surface of the patellar tendon. The prepatellar bursa lies between the subcutaneous tissues and the patella. (From Lormeau C, Cormier G, Sigaux J, et al. Management of septic bursitis. *Joint Bone Spine.* 2019;86[5]:583–588, Fig. 1.)

series of loculated sacs. The deep infrapatellar bursa is vulnerable to injury from both acute trauma and repeated microtrauma. Acute injuries are caused by direct trauma to the bursa during falls onto the knee (Fig. 9.5) or patellar fracture. Overuse injuries are caused by running on soft or uneven surfaces or being in positions that require crawling and kneeling, such as praying. If inflammation of the deep infrapatellar bursa becomes chronic, calcification may occur.

SIGNS AND SYMPTOMS

Patients with deep infrapatellar bursitis complain of pain and swelling in the anterior knee below the patella that can radiate inferiorly into the surrounding area. Often patients are unable to kneel or walk down stairs. They may also complain of a sharp "catching" sensation with range of motion of the knee, especially on first arising. Infrapatellar bursitis often coexists with arthritis and tendinitis of the knee, which can confuse the clinical picture.

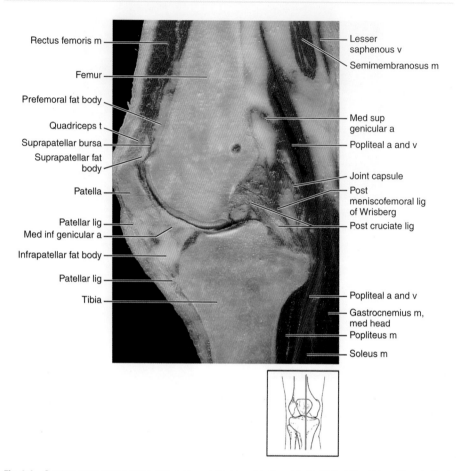

Rectus femoris m

Femur

Prefemoral fat body

Quadriceps t

Suprapatellar bursa

Suprapatellar fat body

Patella

Patellar lig
Med inf genicular a

Infrapatellar fat body

Patellar lig

Tibia

Lesser saphenous v

Semimembranosus m

Med sup genicular a

Popliteal a and v

Joint capsule

Post meniscofemoral lig of Wrisberg

Post cruciate lig

Popliteal a and v

Gastrocnemius m, med head

Popliteus m

Soleus m

Fig. 9.4 Sagittal view of the knee. (From Kang HS, Ahn JM, Resnick D. *MRI of the Extremities*. 2nd ed. Philadelphia: Saunders; 2002:337.)

Physical examination may reveal point tenderness in the anterior knee just below the patella. Swelling and fluid accumulation surrounding the lower patella are often present (see Fig. 9.3). Passive flexion and active resisted extension of the knee reproduce the pain. Sudden release of resistance during this maneuver causes a marked increase in pain. The deep infrapatellar bursa is not as susceptible to infection as is the superficial infrapatellar bursa.

TESTING

Plain radiographs, ultrasound, and magnetic resonance imaging (MRI) of the knee may reveal calcification of the bursa and associated structures, including

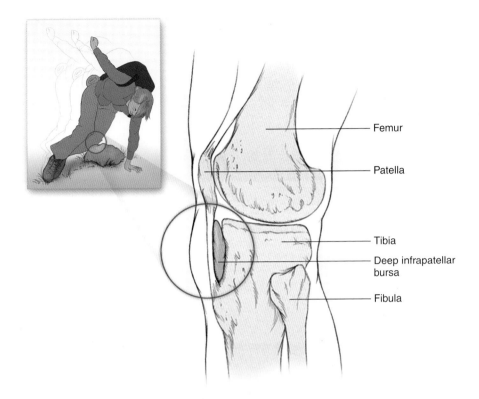

Fig. 9.5   Deep infrapatellar bursitis may result from direct trauma, such as falling on the knee. (From Waldman SD. *Atlas of Common Pain Syndromes*. 4th ed. Philadelphia: Elsevier; 2019: Fig. 115.1.)

the quadriceps tendon, findings consistent with chronic inflammation (Figs. 9.6 and 9.7). MRI and ultrasound imaging is indicated if internal derangement, an occult mass, or a tumor of the knee is suspected as well as to identify other causes of the patient's knee pain (Fig. 9.8). Electromyography can distinguish deep infrapatellar bursitis from femoral neuropathy, lumbar radiculopathy, and plexopathy. The injection technique described later serves as both a diagnostic and a therapeutic maneuver. Antinuclear antibody testing is indicated if collagen vascular disease is suspected. If infection is a possibility, aspiration, Gram stain, and culture of bursal fluid should be performed on an emergency basis.

DIFFERENTIAL DIAGNOSIS

Because of the anatomy of the region, the associated tendons and other bursae of the knee can become inflamed along with the deep infrapatellar bursa, thus confusing the diagnosis. Both the quadriceps tendon and the deep infrapatellar

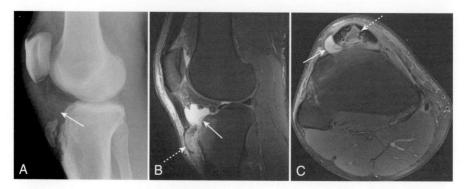

Fig. 9.6 Deep infrapatellar bursitis. Lateral radiograph of a patient with chronic insertional tendinopathy of the patellar tendon with nonfused tibial apophysis. There is soft tissue shadowing deep to the distal patellar tendon *(white arrow)* that partly obliterates the Hoffa fat pad. The sagittal (B) and axial (C) T2-weighted with fat suppression (FST2W) magnetic resonance (MR) images clearly show the high signal intensity (SI) fluid within the deep infrapatellar bursa *(white arrows)*. There is also high SI marrow edema within the unfused apophysis and adjacent tibia *(broken white arrows)*. (From Waldman SD, Campbell RSD. *Imaging of Pain*. Philadelphia: Elsevier.)

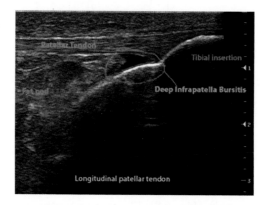

Fig. 9.7 Longitudinal ultrasound image of the knee joint demonstrating deep infrapatellar bursitis. Note the relationship of the bursa to the patellar tendon. (Courtesy Steven Waldman, MD.)

bursa are subject to inflammation from overuse, misuse, or direct trauma. The tendon fibers, called expansions, are vulnerable to strain, and the tendon proper is subject to the development of tendinitis. The suprapatellar, infrapatellar, and prepatellar bursae may also become inflamed with dysfunction of the quadriceps tendon. Anything that alters the normal biomechanics of the knee can result in inflammation of the deep infrapatellar bursa (Table 9.1).

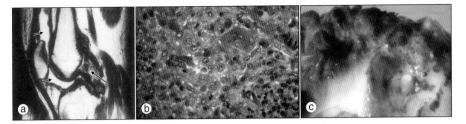

Fig. 9.8 Pigmented villonodular synovitis. (a) Magnetic resonance image of the knee. Short, wide arrows indicate joint effusion in the suprapatellar pouch, and there is a lobulated mass with a typical dark image on T2-weighted scans in the popliteal fossa just below the long arrow. (b) Photomicrograph showing clusters of cells with large pale nuclei and foamy cytoplasm, giant cells, and hemosiderin in the right lower corner. (c) Gross appearance of synovium with pigmented nodules. (From Hochberg M, et al. *Rheumatology*. 7th ed. Philadelphia: Elsevier; 2019: Fig. 214.12.)

TABLE 9.1 ■ Differential Diagnosis of Deep Infrapatellar Bursitis

- Arthritides of the knee
- Patellar abnormalities
- Tendinopathies
- Ligamentous strain
- Avascular necrosis of the knee joint
- Septic arthritis
- Impingement syndromes
- Fractures of the tibial plateau
- Avulsion fractures around the knee
- Iliotibial band inflammation
- Osgood-Schlatter disease
- Complex regional pain syndrome

TREATMENT

A short course of conservative therapy consisting of simple analgesics, nonsteroidal antiinflammatory drugs (NSAIDs) or cyclooxygenase-2 inhibitors, and a knee brace to prevent further trauma is the first step in the treatment of deep infrapatellar bursitis. If patients do not experience rapid improvement, injection of local anesthetic and steroid is a reasonable next step (Fig. 9.9). The use of ultrasound needle guidance will improve the accuracy of needle placement and decrease the incidence of needle-related complications.

Physical modalities, including local heat and gentle range of motion exercises, should be introduced several days after the patient undergoes injection. Vigorous exercises should be avoided because they will exacerbate the patient's symptoms. Simple analgesics and NSAIDs can be used concurrently with this injection technique.

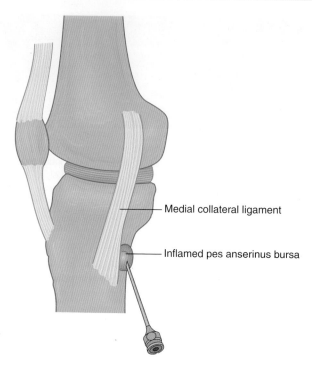

Medial collateral ligament

Inflamed pes anserinus bursa

Fig. 9.9   Injection of local anesthetic and steroid is useful in the management of the pain and swelling associated with deep infrapatellar bursitis. (From Waldman SD. *Atlas of Pain Management Injection Techniques*. 4th ed. St Louis: Elsevier; 2017: Fig. 144-3.)

HIGH-YIELD TAKEAWAYS

- The patient is afebrile, making an acute infectious etiology (e.g., septic arthritis) unlikely.
- The patient's symptomatology is presumably the result of repetitive microtrauma, and physical examination and testing should be focused on the identification of ligamentous injury, acute arthritis, tendinitis, and bursitis.
- The patient has point tenderness over the deep infrapatellar bursa, which is highly suggestive of deep infrapatellar bursitis.
- There is warmth and swelling of the area overlying the deep infrapatellar bursa, suggestive of an inflammatory process.
- The patient's symptoms are unilateral and involve only one joint, which is more suggestive of a local process than a systemic polyarthropathy.

(Continued)

- Sleep disturbance is common and must be addressed concurrently with the patient's pain symptomatology.
- Plain radiographs will provide high-yield information regarding the bony contents of the joint and the identification of fractures or other bony abnormalities of the femur as well as calcification of the bursa and tendons, but ultrasound imaging and MRI will be more useful in identifying soft tissue pathology.

Suggested Readings

Steinbach LS, Stevens KJ. Imaging of cysts and bursae about the knee. *Radiol Clin N Am*. 2013;51(3):433–454.

Waldman SD. Bursitis syndromes of the knee. In: *Pain Review*. 2nd ed. Philadelphia: Elsevier; 2017:306–308.

Waldman SD. Deep infrapatellar bursa injection. In: *Atlas of Pain Management Injection Techniques*. 4th ed. Philadelphia: Elsevier; 2017:533–535.

Waldman SD. Deep infrapatellar bursitis. In: *Waldman's Comprehensive Atlas of Diagnostic Ultrasound of Painful Conditions*. 1st ed. Philadelphia: Wolters Kluwer; 2016:799–804.

Waldman SD, Campbell RSD. Deep infrapatellar bursitis. In: *Imaging of Pain*. 1st ed. Philadelphia: Saunders; 2011:408–410.

Kitty Lee

A 24-Year-Old Optician With Severe Left Anteriomedial Knee Pain

LEARNING OBJECTIVES

- Learn the common causes of knee pain.
- Develop an understanding of the unique anatomy of the knee joint.
- Develop an understanding of the bursae of the knee.
- Develop an understanding of the causes of pes anserine bursitis.
- Develop an understanding of the differential diagnosis of pes anserine bursitis.
- Learn the clinical presentation of pes anserine bursitis.
- Learn how to examine the knee and associated bursae.
- Learn how to use physical examination to identify pes anserine bursitis.
- Develop an understanding of the treatment options for pes anserine bursitis.

Kitty Lee

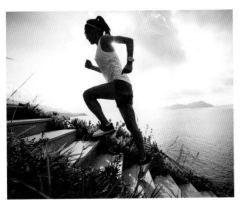

Kitty Lee is a 24-year-old female optician with the chief complaint of, "The inside of my knee hurts." Kitty stated that over the past several weeks, the inside of her left knee really started hurting. She went on to say that the knee pain has really been "messing with my workout." I asked Kitty if she had ever had anything like this before and she said, "My knees were fine until I missed that step. Doctor, do you know that trail in Griffith Park that takes you up to the Hollywood sign?" I told her I did and she went on to tell me that she likes to run up that trail every morning as part of her workout. "So, I was trying to beat my best time and I was really trucking up the hill when I accidently missed a step. I didn't actually fall, but as I caught my balance, I came down funny on my left knee and kind of twisted it."

I asked Kitty what made the pain worse and she said that any walking, going down stairs, putting on her jogging shoes, squatting, or getting on and off the commode all made the pain much worse, and "jogging was completely out of the question." I asked her what made it better and she reported that Advil helped, but it was upsetting her stomach. She noted that icing the knee felt good, but the pain came back as soon as she took off the ice. I asked Kitty about any antecedent knee trauma and she could not remember any. Kitty volunteered that she has having a real hard time getting a good night's sleep. "Doctor, my serious sleeping position is on my left side and even with a pillow between my legs, whenever my right knee puts pressure on my left knee, it wakes me up."

I asked Kitty to point with one finger where it hurt the most. She pointed to her anteriomedial knee just below the joint space on the left (Fig. 10.1).

On physical examination, Kitty was afebrile. Her respirations were 16 and her pulse was 64 and regular. Her blood pressure was 126/80. Kitty's head, eyes, ears, nose, and throat (HEENT) exam was normal, as was her cardiopulmonary examination. Her thyroid was normal. Her abdominal examination revealed no abnormal mass or organomegaly. There was no costovertebral angle (CVA) tenderness. There was no peripheral edema. Her low back examination revealed some tenderness to deep palpation of the paraspinous musculature. Visual inspection of the left medial knee revealed no obvious ecchymosis, but the area appeared a little swollen. The area over the left pes anserine bursa felt warm but did not appear to be infected. The left medial knee felt "boggy" on palpation.

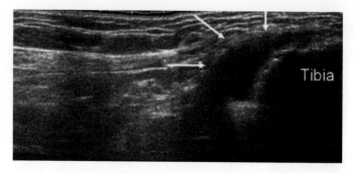

Fig. 10.1   Ultrasound image demonstrating pes anserine bursitis.

There was marked tenderness to palpation over the pes anserine region, with palpation of the area exacerbating Kitty's pain. Range of motion of the knee joint, especially active resisted flexion of the knee joint, caused Kitty to cry out in pain. The right knee examination was normal, as was examination of her major joints. A careful neurologic examination of the upper and lower extremities revealed there was no evidence of peripheral or entrapment neuropathy, and the deep tendon reflexes were normal. I asked Kitty to walk down the hall, where I noted an antalgic gait was present.

Key Clinical Points—What's Important and What's Not
THE HISTORY

- Onset of left knee pain following a jogging injury to the left knee
- Pain localized to the area of the left pes anserine bursa
- Pain made worse by walking, going down stairs, and squatting
- No other specific traumatic events to the knees
- No fever or chills
- Sleep disturbance
- Unable to jog due to persistent left knee pain

THE PHYSICAL EXAMINATION

- The patient is afebrile
- Point tenderness to palpation of the area over the pes anserine bursa
- Palpation of left knee reveals warmth to touch
- The left medial knee is swollen, with "bogginess" over the pes anserine bursa
- No evidence of infection

- Pain on range of motion, especially active resisted flexion of the affected left knee
- An antalgic gait was present

OTHER FINDINGS OF NOTE

- Normal HEENT examination
- Normal cardiovascular examination
- Normal pulmonary examination
- Normal abdominal examination
- Tenderness to deep palpation of the lumbar paraspinous muscles
- No peripheral edema
- Normal upper and lower extremity neurologic examination, motor and sensory examination
- Examinations of joints other than the left knee were normal

 ## What Tests Would You Like to Order?

The following tests were ordered:
- Plain radiographs of the left knee
- Ultrasound of the left knee

TEST RESULTS

The plain radiographs of the left knee reveal mild soft tissue swelling over the medial knee. Ultrasound examination of the left knee revealed pes anserine bursitis (see Fig. 10.1).

 ## Clinical Correlation — Putting It All Together

What is the diagnosis?
- Pes anserine bursitis

The Science Behind the Diagnosis

ANATOMY

The pes anserine bursa lies beneath the pes anserinus (Latin for "goose foot"), which is the insertional conjoined tendons of the sartorius, gracilis, and semitendinous muscles on the medial side of the tibia (Fig. 10.2). This bursa may exist as a single bursal sac or, in some patients, as a multisegmented series of loculated sacs. The pes anserine bursa is susceptible to the development of inflammation

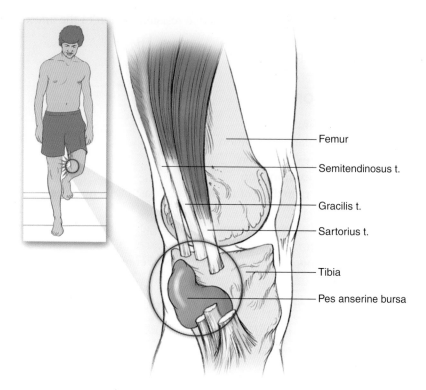

Femur

Semitendinosus t.

Gracilis t.

Sartorius t.

Tibia

Pes anserine bursa

Fig. 10.2   The pes anserine bursa lies beneath the pes anserinus (Latin for "goose foot"), which is the insertional conjoined tendons of the sartorius, gracilis, and semitendinous muscles on the medial side of the tibia. Patients with pes anserine bursitis complain of medial knee pain that is made worse with kneeling or walking down stairs. (From Waldman SD. *Atlas of Common Pain Syndromes*. 4th ed. Philadelphia: Elsevier; 2019: Fig. 118.2.)

from overuse, misuse, or direct trauma. If inflammation of the pes anserine bursa becomes chronic, calcification may occur. Rarely, the pes anserine bursa becomes infected.

CLINICAL SYNDROME

The pes anserine bursa is susceptible to the development of inflammation from overuse, misuse, or direct trauma. If inflammation of the pes anserine bursa becomes chronic, calcification may occur. Rarely, the pes anserine bursa becomes infected. With trauma to the medial knee, the medial collateral ligament is often involved, along with the pes anserine bursa. This broad, flat, bandlike ligament runs from the medial condyle of the femur to the medial aspect of the shaft of the tibia, where it attaches just above the groove of the semimembranosus muscle; it also attaches to the edge of the medial semilunar cartilage. The medial collateral

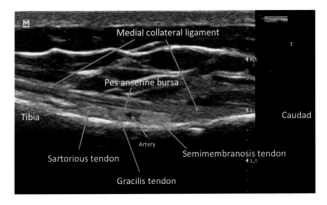

Fig. 10.3 Ultrasound image of the knee joint demonstrating the pes anserine bursa lying beneath the pes anserine tendon. (From Waldman SD. *Atlas of Common Pain Syndromes*. 4th ed. Philadelphia: Elsevier; 2019: Fig. 118.4.)

ligament is crossed at its lower part by the tendons of the sartorius, gracilis, and semitendinosus muscles (Fig. 10.3).

SIGNS AND SYMPTOMS

Patients with pes anserine bursitis present with pain over the anterior medial knee just below the joint and increased pain on active resisted flexion, passive valgus, and external rotation of the knee (Fig. 10.4). Activity, especially involving flexion and external rotation of the knee, makes the pain worse, whereas rest and heat provide some relief. Often, patients are unable to kneel or walk down stairs (see Fig. 10.1). The pain of pes anserine bursitis is constant and is characterized as aching; it may interfere with sleep. Coexistent bursitis, tendinitis, arthritis, or internal derangement of the knee may confuse the clinical picture after trauma to the knee.

Physical examination may reveal point tenderness in the anterior knee just below the medial knee joint at the tendinous insertion of the pes anserine (Fig. 10.5). Swelling and fluid accumulation surrounding the bursa are often present (Fig. 10.6). Active resisted flexion of the knee reproduces the pain. Sudden release of resistance during this maneuver causes a marked increase in pain.

TESTING

Plain radiographs and ultrasound imaging of the knee may reveal degenerative changes and calcification of the bursa and associated structures, including the pes anserine tendon, findings consistent with chronic inflammation (Fig. 10.7). Magnetic resonance imaging (MRI) and ultrasound imaging are indicated if

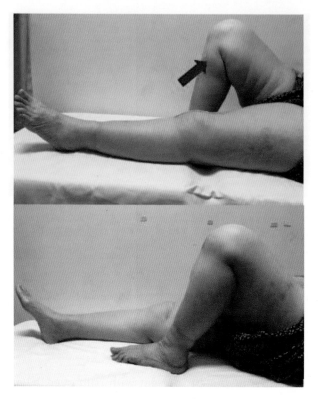

Fig. 10.4   The location of tenderness in pes anserine bursitis *(red arrow).* (From Kamudin NAF, Rani RA, Yahaya NHM. Pes anserine syndrome in post knee arthroplasty. A rare case report. *J Clin Orthop Trauma.* 2020;11[1]:171–174, Fig. 3.)

internal derangement, an occult mass, or a tumor of the knee is suspected (Figs. 10.8 and 10.9). Electromyography can distinguish pes anserine bursitis from neuropathy, lumbar radiculopathy, and plexopathy. Injection of the pes anserine bursa with local anesthetic and steroid may serve as both a diagnostic and a therapeutic maneuver.

DIFFERENTIAL DIAGNOSIS

Pes anserine spurs may coexist with pes anserine bursitis, thus confusing the clinical picture (see Fig. 10.7). Because of the unique anatomic relationships present in the medial knee, it is often difficult to make an accurate clinical diagnosis that identifies the structure responsible for the patient's pain. MRI and ultrasound imaging can rule out medial knee lesions that may require surgical intervention, such as tears of the medial meniscus (Fig. 10.10). Anything that alters the normal biomechanics of the knee can result in inflammation of the pes anserine bursa.

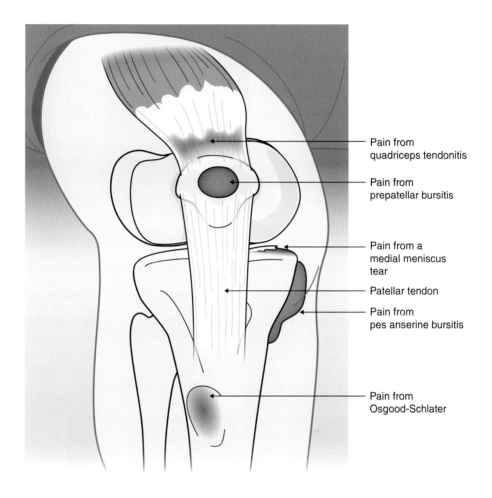

Pain from
quadriceps tendonitis

Pain from
prepatellar bursitis

Pain from a
medial meniscus
tear

Patellar tendon

Pain from
pes anserine bursitis

Pain from
Osgood-Schlater

Fig. 10.5 The pain of pes anserine bursitis is localized to the anterior medial knee.

TREATMENT

A short course of conservative therapy consisting of simple analgesics, nonsteroidal antiinflammatory drugs (NSAIDs) or cyclooxygenase-2 inhibitors, and a knee
brace to prevent further trauma is the first step in the treatment of pes anserine
bursitis. If patients do not experience rapid improvement, injection of the pes
anserine bursa with local anesthetic and steroid is a reasonable next step
(Fig. 10.11). The use of ultrasound needle guidance will improve the accuracy of
needle placement and decrease the incidence of needle-related complications. A
recent large series of 169 cases demonstrated the efficacy of cupping in the treatment of patients suffering from pes anserine bursitis (Fig. 10.12).

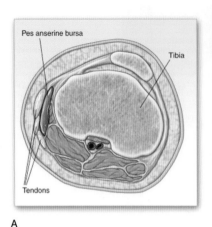

A

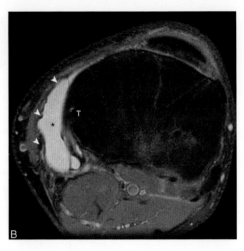

B

Fig. 10.6 Drawing illustrating pes anserine bursitis. (A) This axial view shows the anserine bursa *(blue)* located between the medial aspect of the tibia and the tendons, forming the pes anserinus (from anterior to posterior: sartorius, gracilis, and semitendinosus). (B) Axial proton density (PD)—weighted image with fat suppression shows a fluid collection *(asterisk)* located between the pes anserine bursitis *(arrowheads)* and the surface of the medial tibial condyle *(T)*, consistent with anserine bursitis. (From Marra MD, Crema MD, Chung M, et al. MRI features of cystic lesions around the knee. *Knee.* 2008;15:423—438.)

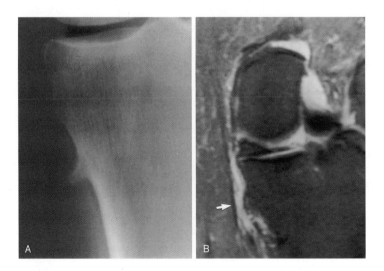

Fig. 10.7 Pes anserine spurs. In this 65-year-old woman with a history of pes anserine bursitis, a conventional radiograph (A) reveals a small excrescence in the medial portion of the tibia. On a coronal, fat-suppressed, fast spin-echo magnetic resonance image (B), fluid of high signal intensity *(arrow)* is seen about the bone outgrowth. (From Resnick D. *Diagnosis of Bone and Joint Disorders.* 4th ed. Philadelphia: Saunders; 2002:3898.)

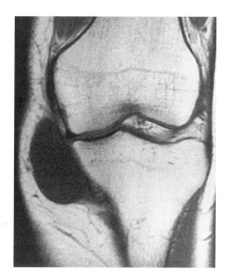

Fig. 10.8 Pes anserinus ganglion cyst (bursitis). Magnetic resonance image shows a large, fluid-filled mass adjacent to the anteromedial portion of the tibia. (From Resnick D. Diagnosis of bone and joint disorders. 4th ed. Philadelphia: Saunders; 2002.)

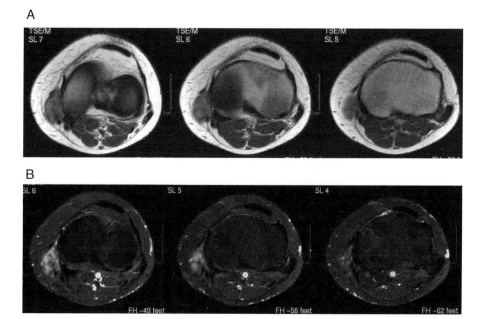

Fig. 10.9 Magnetic resonance imaging (MRI) of a giant cell tumor of the tendinous insertion of the pes anserinus. (A) T1WI + Gad: contiguous images, superior to inferior. The mass enhances and is hyperintense to muscle. The lesion abuts the tendons of sartorius muscle (anteriorly) and gracilis (posteriorly). (B) T1WI + Gad with FS: contiguous images, superior to inferior. The enhancement of the mass is more conspicuous. *T1W1*, weighted image; *Gad*, gadolinium. (From Solomou A, Kraniotis P. Giant cell tumor of the tendon sheath of the tendinous insertion in pes anserinus. *Radiol Case Rep.* 2017;12[2]:353–356, Fig. 3.)

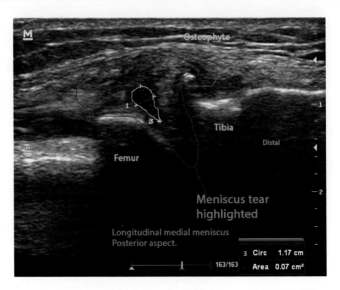

Fig. 10.10   Longitudinal ultrasound image demonstrating a tear of the medial meniscus in a patient with medial knee pain.

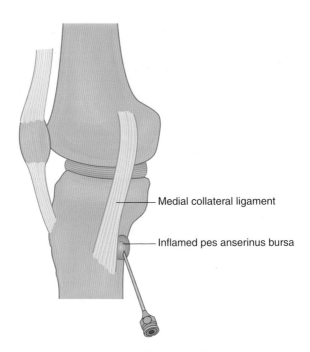

Fig. 10.11   Injection of the pes anserine bursa with local anesthetic and steroid may provide symptomatic relief of the pain and swelling associated with pes anserine bursitis. (From Waldman SD. *Atlas of Pain Management Injection Techniques*. 4th ed. St Louis: Elsevier; 2017, Fig. 144-3.)

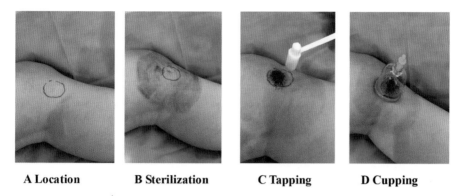

| A Location | B Sterilization | C Tapping | D Cupping |

Fig. 10.12 Bloodletting with plum-blossom needle and cupping for pes anserinus bursitis. (From Cai S, Jin Y, Zhang W, et al. Bloodletting-cupping for 169 cases of pes anserinus myotenositis. *World J Acupunct Moxibust*. 2019;29[3]:231–234, Fig. 1.)

Physical modalities, including local heat and gentle range of motion exercises, should be introduced several days after the patient undergoes injection. Vigorous exercises should be avoided because they will exacerbate the patient's symptoms. Simple analgesics and NSAIDs can be used concurrently with this injection technique.

HIGH-YIELD TAKEAWAYS

- The patient is afebrile, making an acute infectious etiology (e.g., septic arthritis) unlikely.
- The patient's symptomatology is the result of acute trauma and physical examination, and testing should be focused on the identification of ligamentous injury, acute arthritis, tendinitis, and bursitis.
- The patient has point tenderness over the pes anserine bursa, which is highly suggestive of pes anserine bursitis.
- There is warmth and swelling of the area overlying the pes anserine bursa, suggestive of an inflammatory process.
- The patient's symptoms are unilateral and involve only one joint, which is more suggestive of a local process than a systemic polyarthropathy.
- Sleep disturbance is common and must be addressed concurrently with the patient's pain symptomatology.
- Plain radiographs will provide high-yield information regarding the bony contents of the joint and the identification of fractures or other bony abnormalities of the femur as well as calcification of the bursa and tendons, but ultrasound imaging and MRI will be more useful in identifying soft tissue pathology.

Suggested Readings

Maheshwari AV, Muro-Cacho CA, Pitcher Jr JD. Pigmented villonodular bursitis/ diffuse giant cell tumor of the pes anserine bursa: a report of two cases and review of literature. *Knee*. 2007;14(5):402−407.

Steinbach LS, Stevens KJ. Imaging of cysts and bursae about the knee. *Radiol Clin N Am*. 2013;51(3):433−454.

Waldman SD. Bursitis syndromes of the knee. In: *Pain Review*. 2nd ed. Philadelphia: Elsevier; 2017:306−308.

Waldman SD. Pes anserine bursa injection. In: *Atlas of Pain Management Injection Techniques*. 4th ed. Philadelphia: Elsevier; 2017:536−539.

Waldman SD. Pes anserine bursitis. In: *Waldman's Comprehensive Atlas of Diagnostic Ultrasound of Painful Conditions*. 1st ed. Philadelphia: Wolters Kluwer; 2016:805−809.

Saoirse O'Sullivan

A 14-Year-Old Competitive Irish Dancer With Severe Left Anterior Knee Pain

- Learn the common causes of knee pain.
- Develop an understanding of the unique anatomy of the knee joint.
- Develop an understanding of the bursae of the knee.
- Develop an understanding of the causes of Osgood-Schlatter disease.
- Develop an understanding of the differential diagnosis of Osgood-Schlatter disease.
- Learn the clinical presentation of Osgood-Schlatter disease.
- Learn how to examine the knee, associated bursae, and the tibial tuberosity.
- Learn how to use physical examination to identify Osgood-Schlatter disease.
- Develop an understanding of the treatment options for Osgood-Schlatter disease.

Saoirse O'Sullivan

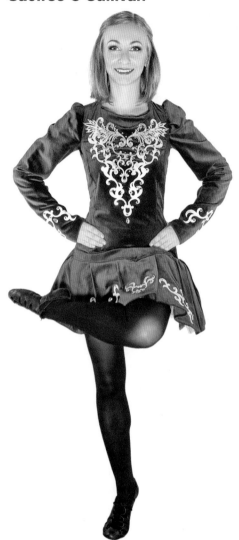

Saoirse O'Sullivan is a 14-year-old competitive Irish dancer with the chief complaint of "There's a painful bump below my left knee and it's embarrassing." Saoirse stated that over the past several months, she has noticed a bump just below her left knee that has gotten bigger and bigger. Saoirse stated that over the past month, the pain has become so painful that it is difficult for her to practice for her Irish dance competitions. "Doctor, dancing is the most important thing in my life, and I want to get rid of this ugly bump on my knee. It's hugely embarrassing to be up on stage and having everyone look at it. The pain is bad, too, but that bump just makes me want to cry." I reassured her that I understood how she felt and would do everything I could to get it better. "So, Saoirse, have you ever had anything like this before?" She said, "No, Doctor, never." "Any previous knee injuries?" I asked, and she again replied, "No, never."

I asked Saoirse what made the pain worse and she said that dancing really made it hurt. I asked, "Anything else?" She said that any walking, going up and down stairs, and walking up the hill on her way to school—really any activity—made the pain worse. I asked her what made it better and she said that the pain got a lot better when she rested the knee, and she thought that Nuprin helped, but she was not allowed to take it when at school. She also thought that the heating pad felt good, but she didn't like the way it made the bump so red. Saoirse denied significant sleep disturbance.

I asked Saoirse to point with one finger to show me where it hurt the most and she immediately pointed to the obviously enlarged tibial tuberosity (Fig. 11.1).

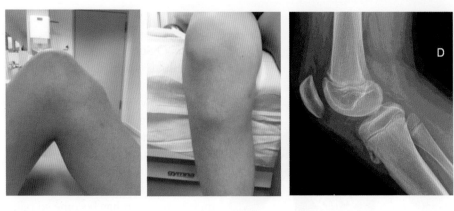

Fig. 11.1 Clinical appearance and radiographic findings in a patient with Osgood-Scholatter disease. (From Nührenbörger C, Gaulrapp H. Morbus Osgood Schlatter. *Sports Orthop Traumatol*. 2018;34 [4]:393–395 [Fig.1].)

On physical examination, Saoirse was afebrile. Her respirations were 16 and her pulse was 70 and regular. Her blood pressure was 106/72. Saoirse's head, eyes, ears, nose, throat (HEENT) exam was normal, as was her cardiopulmonary examination. Her thyroid was normal. Her abdominal examination revealed no abnormal mass or organomegaly. There was no costovertebral angle (CVA) tenderness. There was no peripheral edema. Her low back examination was normal. Visual inspection of the left knee revealed an enlarged tibial tuberosity on the left, which felt warm to touch but did not appear to be infected. The range of motion of the left knee was within normal limits. There was marked tenderness to palpation over the left tibial tuberosity, with the palpation of the area reproducing Saoirse's pain. The right knee examination was normal, as was examination of her major joints. A careful neurologic examination of the upper and lower extremities revealed there was no evidence of peripheral or entrapment neuropathy, and the deep tendon reflexes were normal.

Key Clinical Points—What's Important and What's Not
THE HISTORY

- Gradual enlargement of the left tibial tuberosity
- Increase in pain in the area of the left tibial tuberosity
- Unhappy with cosmetic appearance of left knee
- Onset of left knee pain following Irish dancing
- Pain localized to the area of the left prepatellar region
- Pain associated with swelling of the affected knee

- Pain made worse by dance, walking, stairs, and walking up grades
- No other specific traumatic event to the area identified
- No fever or chills
- Unable to participate in competitive Irish dancing

THE PHYSICAL EXAMINATION

- The patient is afebrile
- Obvious enlargement of the left tibial tuberosity
- Point tenderness to palpation of the area over the tibial tuberosity
- Palpation of left knee reveals warmth to touch
- No evidence of infection
- Normal range of motion of the affected knee

OTHER FINDINGS OF NOTE

- Normal HEENT examination
- Normal cardiovascular examination
- Normal pulmonary examination
- Normal abdominal examination
- No tenderness to deep palpation of the lumbar paraspinous muscles
- No peripheral edema
- Normal upper and lower extremity neurologic examination, motor and sensory examination
- Examinations of joints other than the left knee were normal

What Tests Would You Like to Order?

The following tests were ordered:
- Plain radiographs of the left knee
- Ultrasound of the left knee
- Magnetic resonance imaging (MRI) of the left knee

TEST RESULTS

The plain radiographs of the left knee reveal a prominent tibial tuberosity with an ossicle proximal to the tubercle (see Fig. 11.1). Ultrasound examination of the left knee revealed prepatellar bursitis and plica formation. Osteophyte and patella-femoral degenerative changes are noted (Fig. 11.2). MRI reveals a prominent tibial tuberosity with marrow edema and associated thickening of the patellar tendon (Fig. 11.3).

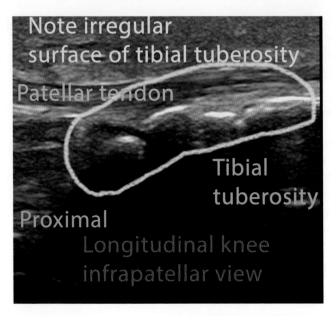

Fig. 11.2 Logitudinal infrapatellar ultrasound image demonstrating the insertion of the patellar tendon on the tibial tuberosity with characteristic bony changes of the tuberosity commonly seen in Osgood-Schlatter disease.

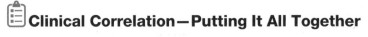 **Clinical Correlation—Putting It All Together**

What is the diagnosis?
- Osgood-Schlatter disease

The Science Behind the Diagnosis

ANATOMY

The quadriceps tendon is made up of fibers from the four muscles that comprise the quadriceps muscle: the vastus lateralis, the vastus intermedius, the vastus medialis, and the rectus femoris (Fig. 11.4). These muscles are the primary extensors for lower extremity at the knee. The tendons of these muscles converge and unite to form a single, exceedingly strong tendon. The patella functions as a sesamoid bone within the quadriceps tendon, with fibers for tendon expanding around the patella and forming the medial and lateral patella retinacula, which help strengthen the knee joint. These fibers are called expansions and are subject to strain; the tendon proper is subject to the development of tendinitis. These fibers continue as the patellar tendon, which originates at the superior pole of the patella, and is comprised of

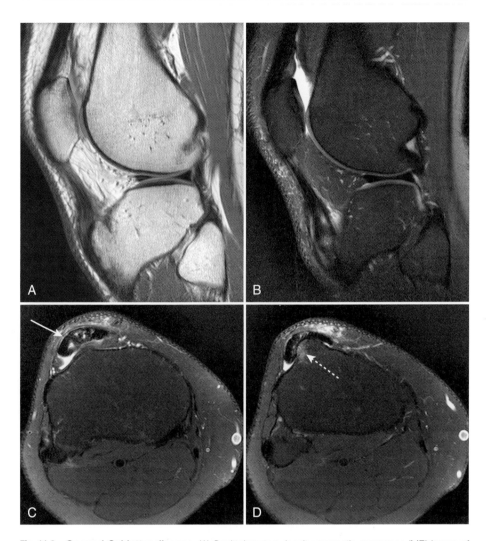

Fig. 11.3 Osgood-Schlatter disease. (A) Sagittal proton density magnetic resonance (MR) image of a young adult with anterior knee pain. The tibial tuberosity is prominent as a result of adolescent Osgood-Schlatter disease. (B) The sagittal T2-weighted with fat suppression (FST2W) MR image shows associated increased signal intensity (SI) within a thickened distal patellar tendon. The axial FST2W MR images (C, D) also show the tendon changes *(white arrow)* and the marrow edema in the tibial tuberosity *(broken white arrow)* due to chronic insertional tendinopathy. (From Waldman SD, Campbell RSD. *Imaging of Pain*. Philadelphia: Saunders; 2011: Fig. 155.2.)

fibers from the quadriceps tendon, which pass over the top of and on each side of the patella to ultimately insert on the tibial tuberosity (see Fig. 11.4). It is the attachment of the patellar tendon at the tibial tuberosity that is the site of pathogenesis of Osgood-Schlatter disease.

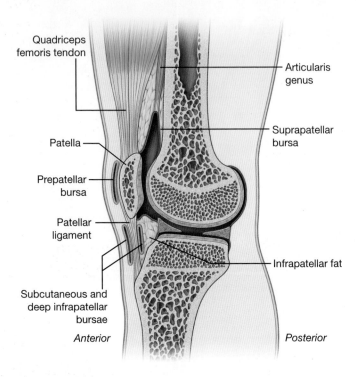

Quadriceps femoris tendon

Articularis genus

Suprapatellar bursa

Patella

Prepatellar bursa

Patellar ligament

Infrapatellar fat

Subcutaneous and deep infrapatellar bursae

Anterior

Posterior

Fig. 11.4   The quadriceps tendon is made up of fibers from the four muscles that comprise the quadriceps muscle: the vastus lateralis, the vastus intermedius, the vastus medialis, and the rectus femoris. (From Waldman SD. *Pain Review*. 2nd ed. Philadelphia: Elsevier; 2017: Fig. 84-1.)

CLINICAL SYNDROME

Originally described by Osgood and Schlatter in 1903, Osgood-Schlatter disease, which is also known as apophysitis of the tibial tubercle, is a common cause of anterior knee pain that can usually be diagnosed on the basis of a targeted history and physical examination. The pathogenesis of Osgood-Schlatter disease is thought to be due to excessive repetitive force on the tibial tuberosity by traction of the patellar tendon from quadriceps muscle contraction. This chronic traction creates inflammation of the ossification center of the proximal tibia with resultant avulsion of the secondary ossification center. If the traction injury continues, a nonunion of the avulsed bony fragments results (Fig. 11.5).

Occurring more commonly in adolescent boys, Osgood-Schlatter disease presents with the complaint of anterior knee pain that is made worse with squatting, running, jumping, sports, going up and down stairs, and Irish and Scottish dancing. The pain of Osgood-Schlatter disease is bilateral approximately 50% of the

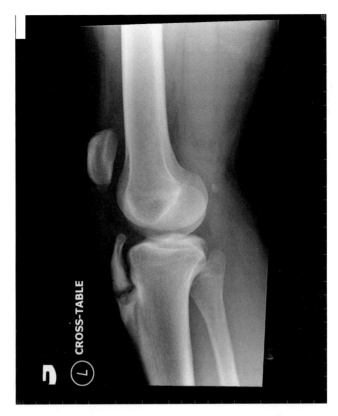

Fig. 11.5 X-ray left knee on initial presentation. Large ossicle, 4 cm in length, seen at the tibial tubercle, separated from the tubercle. The ossicle is seen indenting into the joint space. (From Talawadekar GD, Mostofi B, Housden P. Unusually large sized bony ossicle in Osgood Schlatter disease. *Eur J Radiol Extra*. 2009;69[1]:e37—e39 [Fig 1].)

time, although one side may be worse than the other. The pain characteristically improves with rest and exacerbates with activity. There is rarely a history of significant identifiable trauma.

Although the disease can affect all ages, most cases occur in adolescents, with a peak incidence at approximately 13 years of age. Boys and men are affected two to three times more often than are girls and women, although some investigators believe that the number of female cases is on the rise as a result of increased female participation in competitive sports. The pain and functional disability associated with Osgood-Schlatter disease are bilateral in 25% to 30% of patients, and one side often has more severe symptoms. Osgood-Schlatter disease is usually the result of overuse or misuse of the knee joint caused by running, jumping, or overtraining on hard surfaces, as well as any other activities that require repetitive quadriceps contraction. Competitive sports most often implicated in the development of Osgood-Schlatter disease include soccer,

---

BOX 11.1 ■ Sports Commonly Associated With Osgood-Schlatter Disease

- Soccer
- Gymnastics
- Basketball
- Baseball
- Track
- Hockey
- Ballet
- Irish—style line dancing
- Scottish Highland—style dancing

---

gymnastics, basketball, ballet, track, hockey, baseball, and Irish and Scottish Highland—style dancing (Box 11.1).

SIGNS AND SYMPTOMS

On physical examination, the finding of point tenderness over the tibial tubercle is pathognomonic for Osgood-Schlatter disease. Enlargement of the tibial tubercle is invariably present, with consistently reproducible pain with direct palpation, resisted knee extension, and jumping, which causes the quadriceps muscle to contract and place traction via the quadriceps tendon, expansions, and patellar tendon on the tibial tuberosity. Moderate rubor may be present around the tibial tuberosity, but there will be no obvious joint effusion, as is seen with bursitis of the knee. The range of motion of the knee is within normal limits, as is the neurovascular examination. If the disease is left untreated, atrophy of the quadriceps muscle may result. Box 11.2 provides the clinician with a differential diagnosis for Osgood-Schlatter disease. It is important to rule out other diseases that may cause permanent damage to the knee if left untreated.

TESTING

Plain radiographs are indicated in all patients who present with knee pain and who are suspected of suffering from Osgood-Schlatter disease (Figs. 11.6 and 11.7). MRI of the knee is indicated if Osgood-Schlatter disease is suspected because it readily detects any disorder of the patellar tendon as well as the condition of the tibial tuberosity (Figs. 11.8 and 11.9; see Fig. 11.7). Ultrasound imaging may also provide beneficial information regarding the vascularity and integrity of the patellar tendons and the presence of tibial tuberosity abnormalities (see Fig. 11.2). Bone scan may be useful to identify occult stress fractures involving the joint, especially if trauma has occurred.

> ### BOX 11.2 ■ Differential Diagnosis for Osgood-Schlatter Disease
>
> Sinding-Larson-Johansson syndrome
> Legg-Perthes disease
> Jumper's knee
> Superficial infrapatellar bursitis
> Deep infrapatellar bursitis
> Prepatellar bursitis
> Septic arthritis
> Cellulitis
> Quadriceps tendinopathy
> Chondromalacia patellae
> Patellar tendonitis
> Osteogenic sarcoma
> Soft tissue malignancy
> Accessory ossicles
> Synovitis
> Tibial plateau fractures
> Anterior cruciate ligament injuries
> Osteomyelitis of the patella
> Osteomyelitis of the tibia
> Hoffa syndrome
> Foreign body
> Synovial plica injury
> Tibial tubercle fracture
> Proximal tibiofibular joint disorders
> Patellofemoral joint disorders

Based on the patient's clinical presentation, additional testing may be indicated, including a complete blood count, erythrocyte sedimentation rate, and antinuclear antibody testing.

DIFFERENTIAL DIAGNOSIS

Osgood-Schlatter disease is a repetitive stress disorder that is a distinct clinical entity from tendinitis of the patellar tendons or quadriceps expansion syndrome. However, such tendinitis, bursitis, and other painful conditions that affect the anterior knee may coexist with Osgood-Schlatter disease and may confuse the clinical picture. Diseases that may mimic Osgood-Schlatter diseases are listed in Box 11.2. Quadriceps expansion syndrome has a predilection for the medial side of the superior pole of the patella. The quadriceps tendon is also subject to acute calcific tendinitis, which may coexist with acute strain injuries and the more chronic changes of Osgood-Schlatter disease. Calcific tendinitis of the quadriceps has a characteristic radiographic appearance of whiskers on the anterosuperior patella. The suprapatellar, infrapatellar, and prepatellar

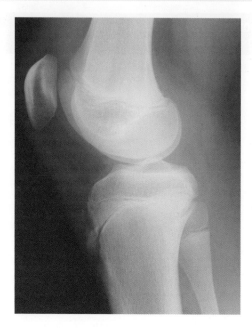

Fig. 11.6   Lateral radiograph of an adolescent with anterior knee pain, demonstrating fragmentation of the tibial tuberosity caused by Osgood-Schlatter disease. (From Waldman SD, Campbell RSD. *Imaging of Pain*. Philadelphia: Elsevier.)

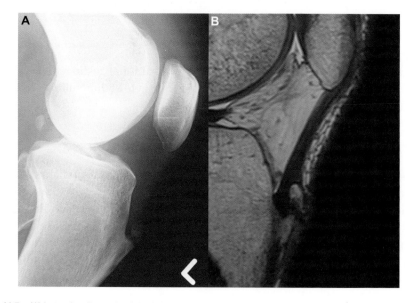

Fig. 11.7   (A) Lateral radiograph of the left knee of the illustrated case shows a prominent tibial tuberosity and ossicle proximal to the tubercle. (B) Magnetic resonance imaging (sagittal, T2-weighted image) shows that the tubercle and ossicle are at the anterior aspect of the patellar tendon. (From Lui TH. Endoscopic management of Osgood-Schlatter disease. *Arthr Tech*. 2016;5[1]:e121−e125 [Fig. 1].)

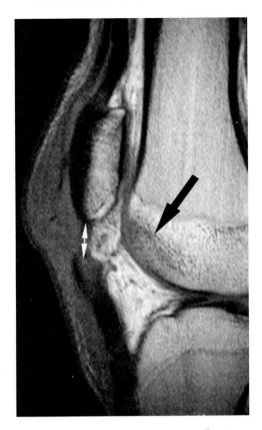

Fig. 11.8 A 26-year-old male long-jumper with full-thickness rupture of the infrapatellar tendon at its patellar attachment. Sagittal T1-weighted magnetic resonance imaging (MRI) of the knee elegantly demonstrating the tendon gap *(white arrow)*. Note also the loss of marrow signal within the femoral trochlea consistent with associated marrow edema *(black arrow)*. (From Peace KAL, Lee JC, Healy J. Imaging the infrapatellar tendon in the elite athlete. *Clin Radiol*. 2006;61[7]:570–578 [Fig. 8].)

bursae also may become inflamed with dysfunction of the quadriceps tendon. Hoffa syndrome, which is a disease affecting the infrapatellar fat pad, may also coexist with Osgood-Schlatter disease.

TREATMENT

Initial treatment of the pain and functional disability associated with Osgood-Schlatter disease includes a combination of nonsteroidal antiinflammatory drugs or cyclooxygenase-2 inhibitors and rest, with the patient avoiding activities that involve contraction of the quadriceps mechanism. The use of therapeutic cold may also provide symptom relief. Gentle physical therapy consisting of stretching of the quadriceps mechanism and the

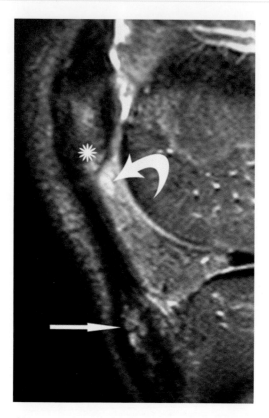

Figure 11.9 A 13-year-old boy with Osgood-Schlatter syndrome. Sagittal T2-weighted gradient echo showing expansion of the distal infrapatellar tendon, which contains areas of intermediate signal due to the nonunited fragmented displaced tibial tubercle apophysis *(arrow)*. Note also the presence of marrow edema within the inferior pole of the patella *(asterisk)* and adjacent fat pad *(curved arrow)*. (From Peace KAL, Lee JC, Healy J. Imaging the infrapatellar tendon in the elite athlete. *Clin Radiol.* 2006;61[7]:570–578 [Fig. 11].)

opposing hamstring muscles should be implemented as the patient's symptoms allow. A nighttime splint and knee pads to protect the knee, as well as the use of an infrapatellar strap during activity, may also help relieve symptoms. For patients who do not respond to these treatment modalities, injection of the tibial tuberosity with local anesthetic and steroid is a reasonable next step. The use of ultrasound needle guidance will improve the accuracy of needle placement and decrease the incidence of needle-related complications.

If the foregoing modalities fail to relieve the patient's symptoms, some experts recommend complete rest of the affected knee by application of a cast for 4 to 6 weeks. In recalcitrant cases, excision of the tibial tuberosity and associated ossicles may be required.

HIGH-YIELD TAKEAWAYS

- The patient is afebrile, making an acute infectious etiology (e.g., septic arthritis) unlikely.
- The patient's symptomatology is the result of acute trauma and physical examination, and testing should be focused on the identification of ligamentous injury, acute arthritis, tendinitis, and bursitis.
- The patient has point tenderness over the tibial tuberosity, which is highly suggestive of Osgood-Schlatter disease.
- There is warmth and swelling of the area overlying the tibial tuberosity, suggestive of an inflammatory process.
- The patient's symptoms are unilateral and involve only one joint, which is more suggestive of a local process than a systemic polyarthropathy.
- Sleep disturbance is common and must be addressed concurrently with the patient's pain symptomatology.
- Plain radiographs will provide high-yield information regarding the bony contents of the joint and the identification of fractures or other bony abnormalities of the femur and tibia as well as calcification of the bursa and tendons, but ultrasound imaging and MRI will be more useful in identifying soft tissue pathology.

Suggested Readings

Belhaj K, Meftah S, Lahrabli S, et al. Osgood-Schlatter and patellar instability: fortuitous association or complication? *Ann Phys Rehabil Med.* 2014;57(suppl 1):e275.

Hong E, Kraft MC. Evaluating anterior knee pain. *Med Clin North Am.* 2014;98 (4):697–717.

Talawadekar GD, Mostofi B, Housden P. Unusually large sized bony ossicle in Osgood-Schlatter disease. *Eur J Radiol Extra.* 2009;69(1):e37–e39.

Waldman SD. Bursitis syndromes of the knee. In: *Pain Review.* 2nd ed. Philadelphia: Elsevier; 2017:306–311.

Waldman SD. Osgood-Schlatter disease. In: *Waldman's Comprehensive Atlas of Diagnostic Ultrasound of Painful Conditions.* Philadelphia: Wolters Kluwer; 2016:810–819.

Waldman SD, Campbell RSD. Anatomy: special imaging considerations of the knee. In: *Imaging of Pain.* Philadelphia: Saunders; 2011:367–368.

Waldman SD, Campbell RSD. Osgood-Schlatter disease. In: *Imaging of Pain.* Philadelphia: Saunders; 2011:408–410.

Will Graham

A 24-Year-Old Youth Pastor With Posterior Left Knee Swelling and Pain

- Learn the common causes of knee pain.
- Learn the common causes of Baker cyst.
- Develop an understanding of the anatomy of the popliteal fossa.
- Develop an understanding of the differential diagnosis of Baker cyst.
- Learn the clinical presentation of Baker cyst.
- Learn how to examine the knee.
- Learn how to examine the popliteal fossa.
- Learn how to use physical examination to identify Baker cyst.
- Develop an understanding of the treatment options for Baker cyst.

Will Graham

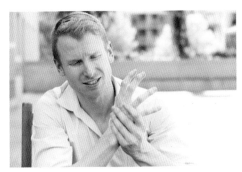

Will Graham is a 24-year-old youth pastor with the chief complaint of, "I've got a bump on the back of my left knee." Will stated that his problems came on over the last month or so. He was leading a youth retreat and they went on a hike, and one of his kids asked what was going on with the back of his knee. He felt the bump on the back of his knee and his first thought was a spider bite. When it didn't get better over the next few days, he began to wonder if he had a tumor on his knee. "Doc, I have so much going on with my rheumatoid arthritis [RA] that I probably don't pay as much attention to things as I should, but this really scared me because it was a little bigger each day and it started to hurt. Then, the crazy thing was that if I was up on my feet a lot, I started getting some numbness and tingling down the front of my leg. I tried using a heating pad, but I thought that it made the bump bigger, so I switched to ice packs. I have been taking Tylenol because my stomach can't take the Motrin." I asked, "What makes it worse?"

"Doc, like I said, if I am on my feet a lot, it gets worse and if I have to squat down to get something out of the bottom drawer of my file cabinet, it feels like the back of my knee is going to pop."

I asked Will how he was sleeping and he shook his head and said, "Not very well. I pray on this, but I'm really scared that I have cancer. I'm really getting worn out." I reassured him that I had a pretty good idea what was going on and it was not likely to be cancer. I told him we would get things figured out. "Just a few more questions and then let's look you over," I said. "Any fever, chills, or other constitutional symptoms such as weight loss, night sweats, etc.?" Will just shook his head no. I asked Will if he had ever had anything like this in the past and he said, "Not really, just the usual ups and down with my RA."

On physical examination, Will was afebrile. His respirations were 16, his pulse was 66 and regular, and his blood pressure was 112/68. Will's head, eyes, ears, nose, throat (HEENT) exam was normal as was his cardiopulmonary examination. His thyroid was normal. His abdominal examination revealed no abnormal mass or organomegaly. There was no costovertebral angle (CVA) tenderness. There was no peripheral edema. His low back examination was unremarkable. Visual inspection of his hands revealed some mild synovitis consistent with his rheumatoid arthritis. There was no ulnar drift. Examination of his left popliteal fossa revealed a firm, tender, cystic mass that was most likely a Baker cyst (Fig. 12.1). There was no rubor, no obvious

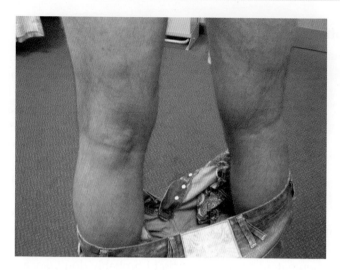

Fig. 12.1 Baker cyst of the left knee. (From Ali F. Clinical examination of the knee. *Orthop Trauma.* 2013;27(1):50–55.)

infection, or bursitis. There was no evidence of thrombophlebitis, and Homans sign was negative. Examination of Will's feet revealed rheumatoid nodules consistent with his rheumatoid arthritis (Fig. 12.2). A careful neurologic examination of the upper extremities was completely normal. Deep tendon reflexes were normal.

Key Clinical Points—What's Important and What's Not

THE HISTORY

- A history of the onset of left posterior knee swelling and pain
- History of rheumatoid arthritis
- No numbness
- No weakness
- No history of previous significant knee pain
- No fever or chills
- Sleep disturbance
- Pain on weightbearing and squatting

THE PHYSICAL EXAMINATION

- The patient is afebrile
- Firm cystic mass in the left popliteal fossa
- Tenderness on palpation of the popliteal mass
- No thrombophlebitis of pseudothrobophebitis

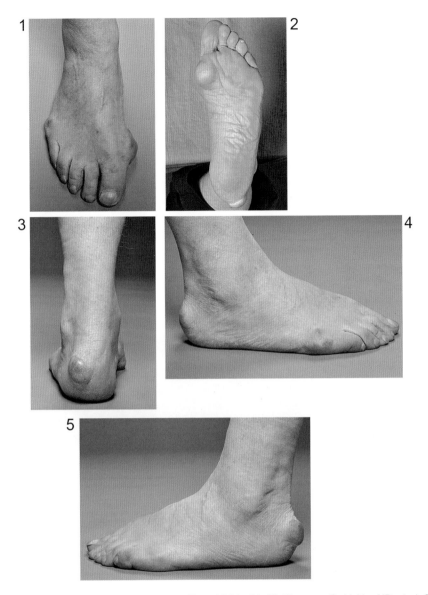

Fig. 12.2 Rheumatoid nodules of the feet. (From McMurrich W, Thomson C, McKay ND, et al. Soft tissue swellings in the foot: rheumatoid nodulosis. *Foot*. 2014:24[1]:37−41 [fig 1−5].)

- Rheumatoid nodules of the feet bilaterally
- Mild synovitis of the hands
- No ulnar drift
- Negative Homans sign
- No obvious bursitis
- No obvious infection

OTHER FINDINGS OF NOTE

- Normal HEENT examination
- Normal cardiovascular examination
- Normal pulmonary examination
- Normal abdominal examination
- No peripheral edema
- Normal upper extremity neurologic examination, motor and sensory examination

 ## What Tests Would You Like to Order?

The following tests were ordered:
- Plain radiographs of the left knee
- Ultrasound of the left knee
- Magnetic resonance imaging (MRI) of the left knee

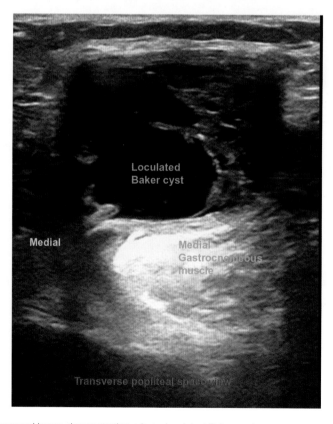

Fig. 12.3   Ultrasound image demonstrating a large loculated Baker cyst.

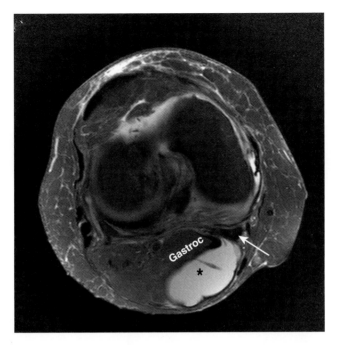

Fig. 12.4   T2-weighted with fat suppression (FST2W) magnetic resonance (MR) image of a Baker cyst in a different patient. The features are identical, with the high signal intensity (SI), fluid-filled cyst *(asterisk)* arising between the gastrocnemius muscle *(Gastroc)* and the semimembranosus tendon *(white arrow)*. (From Waldman SD, Campbell RSD. *Imaging of Pain*. Philadelphia: Elsevier; 2011.)

TEST RESULTS

The plain radiographs of the left knee revealed findings consistent with mild rheumatoid arthritis with no evidence of fracture. Ultrasound examination of the left knee revealed a large Baker cyst (Fig. 12.3). MRI scan of the left knee reveals edema of the tibial insertions of semimembranosus muscle (Fig. 12.4).

Clinical Correlation—Putting It All Together

What is the diagnosis?
■ Baker cyst

The Science Behind the Diagnosis

ANATOMY

The popliteal fossa is posterior to the knee joint. The boundaries of the popliteal fossa are the skin, superficial fascia, and popliteal fascia and the popliteal

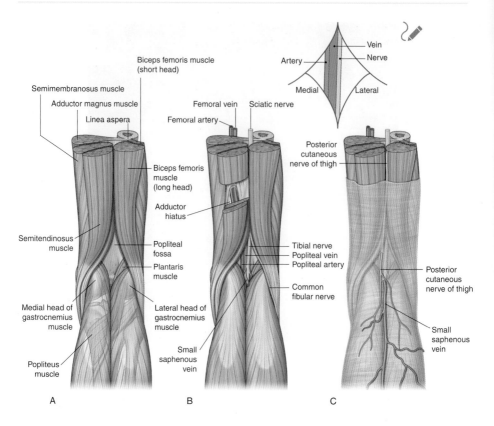

Fig. 12.5 The popliteal fossa. (From Drake R, Vogl AW. *Gray's Anatomy for Students*. 4th ed. Philadelphia: Elsevier; 2020: [fig. 6.83].)

surface of the femur, the capsule of the knee joint, the oblique popliteal ligament, and the fascia of the popliteus muscle. The fossa contains the popliteal artery and vein, the common peroneal and tibial nerves, and the semimembranosus bursa (Fig. 12.5). The knee joint capsule is lined with a synovial membrane that attaches to the articular cartilage and gives rise to a number of bursae, including the suprapatellar, prepatellar, infrapatellar, and semimembranosus bursae, which lie between the medial head of the gastrocnemius muscle, the medial femoral epicondyle, and the semimembranosus tendon. When these bursae and/or the synovial membrane become inflamed, they may overproduce synovial fluid, which can become trapped in saclike cysts because of a one-way valve phenomenon (Fig. 12.6). This occurs commonly in the medial aspect of the popliteal fossa, resulting in the formation of a Baker cyst (see Fig. 12.1).

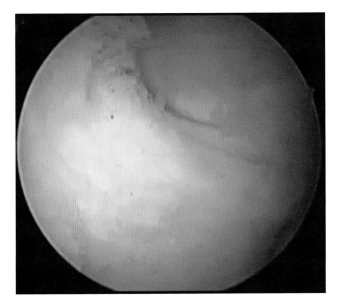

Fig. 12.6 Arthroscopic view of the popliteal fossa showing the classical "one way valve" or "trap door" mechanism of Baker cyst. (From Chahar D, Sreenivasan R, Chawla A, et al. Tuberculosis: an unusual etiology of Baker's cyst. *JAJS*. 2016:3[2]:78–82 [fig 3].)

CLINICAL SYNDROME

Baker cyst, which is also known as popliteal cyst, is a common cause of posterior knee pain and swelling. Baker cyst of the knee is the result of an abnormal accumulation of synovial fluid in the medial aspect of the popliteal fossa, most commonly between the tendons of the medial head of the gastrocnemius and the semimembranosus muscles.

Overproduction of synovial fluid from an inflamed knee joint results in the formation of a cystic sac (Fig. 12.7). This sac often communicates with the knee joint in a one-way valve effect, causing a gradual expansion of the cyst (see Fig. 12.6). Often, a tear of the medial meniscus or tendinitis of the medial hamstring tendon is the inciting factor responsible for the development of a Baker cyst. Patients who suffer from rheumatoid arthritis are especially susceptible to the development of Baker cysts, although any form of arthritis or pathology of the synovium can cause a Baker cyst.

SIGNS AND SYMPTOMS

On physical examination of the patient with a Baker cyst, the clinician may identify a cystic swelling in the medial aspect of the popliteal fossa (see Fig. 12.1). Baker cysts can become quite large, especially in patients who suffer from

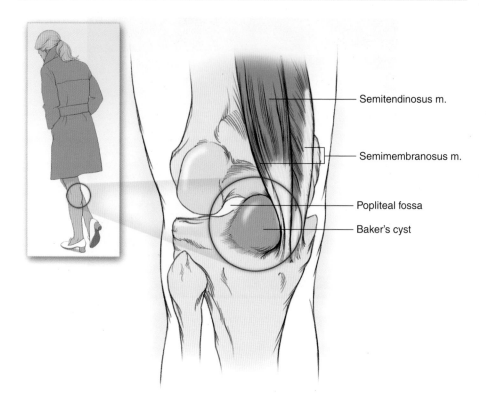

Semitendinosus m.

Semimembranosus m.

Popliteal fossa

Baker's cyst

Fig. 12.7 Patients with Baker cyst often complain of a sensation of fullness or a lump behind the knee. (From Waldman SD. *Atlas of Common Pain Syndromes*. 4th ed. Philadelphia: Elsevier; 2019: Fig. 117.2.)

rheumatoid arthritis. Activity, including squatting, flexing the affected knee, or walking, makes the pain of Baker cyst worse. Rest and heat may provide a modicum of relief. The pain of Baker cyst is constant and is characterized as aching. Sleep disturbance is common. Baker cyst may spontaneously rupture, and resulting rubor and color in the calf that may mimic thrombophlebitis are frequently present (Fig. 12.8). In contradistinction to thrombophlebitis, Homans sign is negative and no cords are palpable. Occasionally, tendinitis of the medial hamstring tendon may be confused with Baker cyst. If the Baker cyst continues to expand, it may impinge on the nerves and arteries that traverse the popliteal fossa (Fig. 12.9).

TESTING

Plain radiographs are indicated in all patients who present with knee pain to aid in the diagnosis and to rule out occult bony pathology (Fig. 12.10). Based on the patient's clinical presentation, additional testing may be indicated, including

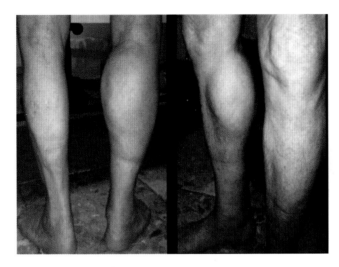

Fig. 12.8 Rupture of a giant Baker cyst mimicking thrombophlebitis. Note the gastrocnemius asymmetry. This physical finding is known as pseudothrombophlebitis. (From Alonso-Gómez N, Pérez-Piqueras A, Martínez-Izquierdo A, Sáinz-González F. Giant Baker' cyst. Differential diagnosis of deep vein thrombosis. *Reumatología Clínica (English Edition)*. 2015;11(3):179—181.)

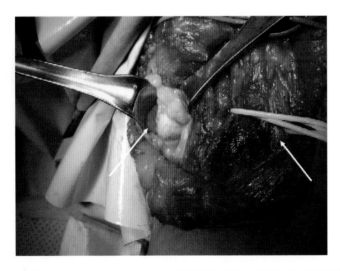

Fig. 12.9 Intraoperative photograph shows thick and whitish Baker cyst found between medial head of gastrocnemius muscle and semimembranosus tendon, which compresses the tibial nerve medially *(arrow)* and displaces the peroneal nerve laterally *(arrow)*. (From Ji J-H, Shafi M, Kim W-Y, et al. Compressive neuropathy of the tibial nerve and peroneal nerve by a Baker's cyst: case report. *Knee*. 2007;14[3]:249—252 [Fig. 3].)

complete blood cell count, sedimentation rate, and antinuclear antibody testing. MRI or ultrasound imaging of the affected area may also confirm the diagnosis and help delineate the presence of other knee bursitis, internal derangement, calcific tendinitis, synovial disease, and tendinopathy (Figs. 12.11, 12.12, and 12.13).

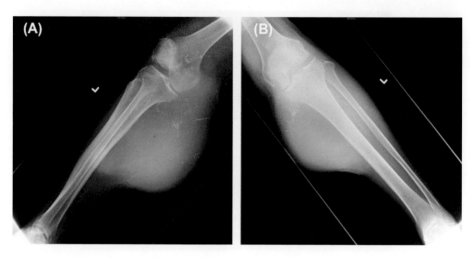

Fig. 12.10 X-rays of the left leg and knee show only mild osteophytes and moderate medial compart-ment narrowing and speckled calcifications at the periphery of the mass. (A) Lateral and (B) anteropos-terior views. (From Hung L-P, Leung Y-F, Lo BA, et al. A huge infected popliteal cyst dissecting into gastrocnemius mimicking calf abscess. *J Orthop Trauma Rehabil.* 2015:19[2]:107−110 [fig 1].)

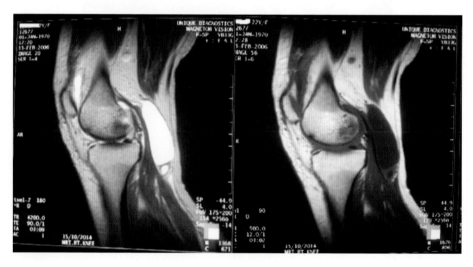

Fig. 12.11 T1- and T2-weighted sagittal magnetic resonance (MR) images revealed a tear in the posterior horn of the medial meniscus along with a well-defined cystic lesion in the gastrocne-mius−semimembranosus bursa appearing hypointense in T1- and hyperintense on T2-weighted images suggestive of a Baker cyst. (From Chahar D, Sreenivasan R, Chawla A, et al. Tuberculosis: an unusual etiology of Baker's cyst. *JAJS.* 2016;3[2]:78−82 [Fig. 1].)

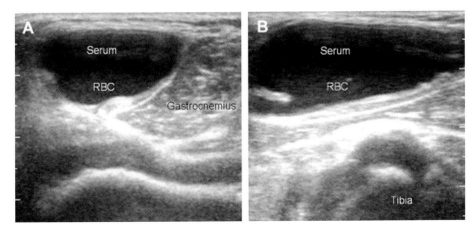

Fig. 12.12 Baker cysts in patient with hemophilia: keeping the patient supine for several minutes is possible to distinguish two layers, serum and red blood cell, both in axial (A) and in sagittal (B) planes. (From Alessi S, Depaoli R, Canepari M, et al. Baker's cyst in pediatric patients: ultrasonographic characteristics. *J Ultrasound.* 2012;15[1]:76–81 [Fig. 5].)

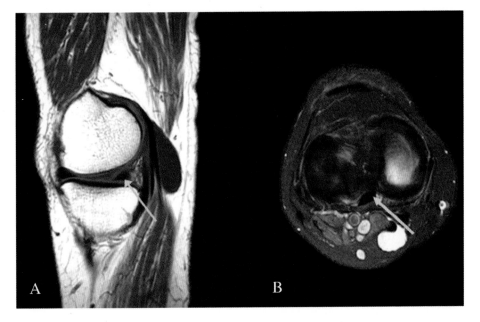

Fig. 12.13 Magnetic resonance imaging (MRI) shows (A) T1-weighted sagittal view posterior medial meniscal tear with cyst in the popliteal area *(arrow)*. (B) T-2 weighted axial view shows cyst communicating with knee joint *(arrow)*. (From Ji J-H, Shafi M, Kim W-Y, et al. Compressive neuropathy of the tibial nerve and peroneal nerve by a Baker's cyst: case report. *Knee.* 2007;14[3]:249–252 [fig 2].)

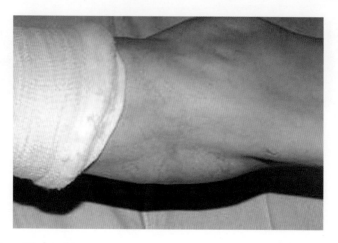

Fig. 12.14 View of the medial aspect of the right knee demonstrates the large swelling in the popliteal fossa, which was subsequently diagnosed on clinical and radiologic testing to be a large right popliteal artery aneurysm. (From Harkin DW, Mohammed O, Khadim M, et al. Rapid expansion of popliteal artery aneurysm after lower limb graduated compression bandaging for varicose ulcer. *EJVES Extra*. 2006;12[1]:6–8 [fig 1].)

DIFFERENTIAL DIAGNOSIS

As mentioned, Baker cysts may rupture spontaneously, thus leading to a misdiagnosis of thrombophlebitis. Occasionally, tendinitis of the medial hamstring or injury to the medial meniscus is confused with Baker cyst. Primary or metastatic tumors in the region, although rare, must also be considered in the differential diagnosis. Care must be taken not to mistake a popliteal artery aneurysm for Baker cyst (Figs. 12.14 and 12.15). Careful palpation of the popliteal fossa should reveal a pulsatile mass if the artery is involved (Table 12.1).

TREATMENT

Although surgery is often required to treat Baker cyst, a short trial of conservative therapy consisting of an elastic bandage and nonsteroidal antiinflammatory drugs or cyclooxygenase-2 inhibitors is warranted. If these conservative measures fail, injection is a reasonable next step.

To inject a Baker cyst, the patient is placed in the prone position with the anterior ankle resting on a folded towel to flex the knee slightly. The middle of the popliteal fossa is identified, and at a point two fingerbreadths medial to and two fingerbreadths below the popliteal crease, the skin is prepared with antiseptic solution. A syringe containing 2 mL of 0.25% preservative-free bupivacaine and 40 mg methylprednisolone is attached to a 2-inch, 22-gauge needle. The needle is

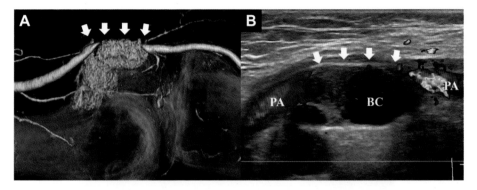

Fig. 12.15 (A) Computed tomography angiography image showing focal narrowing of the popliteal artery *(arrows)* at the right knee. The Baker cyst appears polycystic *(blue masses)* and attached to the popliteal artery. (B) Color Doppler ultrasound image demonstrating flow disturbance in the popliteal artery *(PA)* by the Baker cyst *(BC)*. (From Fujiyoshi K, Minami Y, Tojo T, et al. Lower limb ischemia due to popliteal artery compression by Baker cyst. *J Vasc Surg Cases Innov Tech.* 2018;4[2]:99–101 [Fig. 1].)

TABLE 12.1 ■ Differential Diagnosis of Posterior Knee Swelling and Pain

Baker cyst	Abscess
Popliteal aneurysm	Lymphadnopathy
Sarcoma	Varicosities
Lipoma	Arteriovenous fistula
Metastatic disease	Hematoma
Pigmented villonodular synovitis	Gastrocnemius tear
Ganglion cyst	Planteris muscle tear
Glomus tumor	Synovitis

carefully advanced through the previously identified point at a 45-degree angle from the medial border of the popliteal fossaa, directly toward the Baker cyst. While continuously aspirating, the clinician advances the needle very slowly to avoid trauma to the tibial nerve or popliteal artery or vein. When the cyst is entered, synovial fluid suddenly appears in the syringe. At this point, if no paresthesia is noted in the distribution of the common peroneal or tibial nerve, the contents of the syringe are gently injected. Resistance to injection should be minimal. A pressure dressing is placed over the cyst to prevent fluid reaccumulation. Ultrasound guidance may aid the clinician in needle placement in patients whose anatomic landmarks are difficult to identify, as well as to aid in the drainage of large Baker cysts (Fig. 12.16).

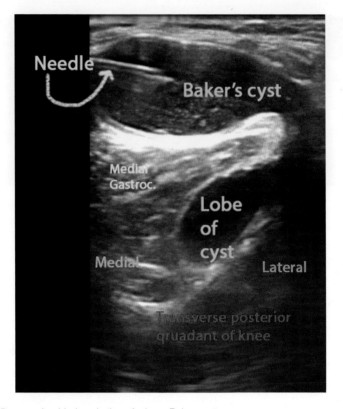

Fig. 12.16 Ultrasound-guided aspiration of a large Baker cyst.

HIGH-YIELD TAKEAWAYS

- The patient is afebrile, making an acute infectious etiology unlikely.
- The patient's symptomatology is thought to be the result of overuse injury to the left popliteal fossa.
- Physical examination and testing should be focused on the identification of diseases that mimic Baker cyst.
- The patient exhibits physical examination findings that are highly suggestive of a Baker cyst.
- The patient's symptoms are unilateral, suggesting a local process rather than a systemic inflammatory process, although the patient has rheumatoid arthritis.
- Plain radiographs will provide high-yield information regarding the bony contents of the joint, but ultrasound imaging and MRI will be more useful in identifying soft tissue pathology that may be responsible for compromise of the contents of the popliteal fossa.

Suggested Readings

Alonso-Gómez N, Pérez-Piqueras A, Martínez-Izquierdo A, et al. Giant Baker cyst. Differential diagnosis of deep vein thrombosis. *Reumatol Clín (English Edition)*. 2015;11(3):179−181.

Drescher MJ, Smally AJ. Thrombophlebitis and pseudothrombophlebitis in the ED. *Am J Emerg Med*. 1997;15(7):683−685.

Marra MD, Crema MD, Chung M, et al. MRI features of cystic lesions around the knee. *Knee*. 2008;15(6):423−438.

Steinbach LS, Stevens KJ. Imaging of cysts and bursae about the knee. *Radiol Clin North Am*. 2013;51(3):433−454.

Torreggiani WC, Al-Ismail K, Munk PL, et al. The imaging spectrum of Baker's (popliteal) cysts. *Clin Radiol*. 2002;57(8):681−691.

Waldman SD. Baker cyst. In: *Waldman's Comprehensive Atlas of Diagnostic Ultrasound of Painful Conditions*. Philadelphia: Wolters Kluwer; 2016:853−860.

Waldman SD. Injection cyst for Baker cyst. In: *Atlas of Pain Management Injection Techniques*. 4th ed. Philadelphia: Elsevier; 2017:556−559.

Waldman SD, Campbell RSD. Baker cyst. In: *Imaging of Pain*. Philadelphia: Saunders; 2011:413−415.

David Pulton

A 26-Year-Old Registered Nurse With Posterolateral Knee Pain

- Learn the common causes of knee pain.
- Learn the common causes of fabella.
- Develop an understanding of the anatomy of the popliteal fossa.
- Develop an understanding of the differential diagnosis of fabella.
- Learn the clinical presentation of fabella.
- Learn how to examine the knee.
- Learn how to examine the popliteal fossa.
- Learn how to use physical examination to identify fabella.
- Develop an understanding of the treatment options for fabella.

David Pulton

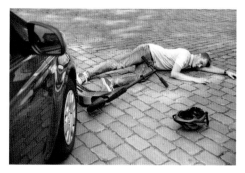

David Pulton is a 26-year-old regis-tered nurse with the chief complaint of, "It feels like I've got gravel in my knee and it really hurts." David stated that his knee symptoms started after he was hit by a car when riding an electric scooter he rented while on vacation. "Doc, I'm really lucky I didn't get killed. That guy really hit me. I was wearing a helmet, but he hit me so hard it knocked the helmet off and I hit my head on the pavement. I hit my head so hard it knocked me out. I was out for over an hour. I woke up in the emergency room at County with the worst headache I have ever had. I had a con-cussion and was off work for about 3 weeks. My head hurt so bad that I was pretty much in bed for a couple of weeks, so I really didn't notice the pain and grating in my left knee until I was up and around." I asked, "Tell me about the knee symptoms." David just shook his head and said, "Doc, this may sound silly, but it feels like there is a piece of gravel in the back of my knee that is rubbing on everything and irritating it. The pain is not severe; it's just always there, down deep, like the back outside of my knee is inflamed. It is really distracting because it never goes away." I asked David what made it worse and he said that stairs were a real killer, as was squatting and being up on his feet during 12-hour shifts. "What makes it better?" I asked. "Doc, I am most comfortable when I have my leg up with a pillow under my knee with the knee slightly flexed. The heating pad helps, as does Motrin."

I asked David how he was sleeping and he said, "Just okay. This whole thing has been very rough, and this knee keeps nagging at me." I reassured David that I would do my best to sort out what was going on and get him better. "Just a few more questions and then let's look you over. Any fever, chills, or other constitu-tional symptoms such as weight loss, night sweats, etc.?" David shook his head no. I asked David if he had ever had any previous left knee injuries and he again shook his head no.

On physical examination, David was afebrile. His respirations were 16, his pulse was 70 and regular, and his blood pressure was 120/70. David's head, eyes, ears, nose, throat (HEENT) exam was normal, as was his cardio-pulmonary examination. His thyroid was normal. His abdominal examina-tion revealed no abnormal mass or organomegaly. There was no costovertebral angle (CVA) tenderness. There was no peripheral edema. His low back examination was unremarkable. Visual inspection of David's knees was unremarkable; specifically, there was no ecchymosis, rubor, or obvious

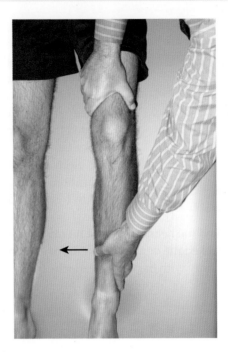

Fig. 13.1   The varus stress test is useful in helping confirm the integrity of the lateral collateral ligament of the knee. (From Waldman SD. *Physical Diagnosis of Pain: An Atlas of Signs and Symptoms*. 3rd ed. St Louis: Elsevier; 2016: Fig. 205-2.)

infection. Examination of his left knee revealed tenderness to palpation of the posterolateral border of the knee. There was a palpable grating sensation with flexion and extension of the left knee. Anterior and posterior drawer signs were negative, as were the valgus and varus stress tests (Fig. 13.1). There was no obvious abnormal mass or bursitis; specifically there was no suggestion of a Baker cyst. There was no evidence of thrombophlebitis or pseudothrombophlebitis, and Homans sign was negative. A careful neurologic examination of the upper extremities was completely normal. Deep tendon reflexes were normal.

Key Clinical Points—What's Important and What's Not

THE HISTORY

- A history of the onset of left posterolateral knee pain after being hit by a car
- A feeling like there is gravel in the knee
- A history of significant concussion
- No numbness
- No weakness

- No history of previous significant knee pain
- No fever or chills
- Sleep disturbance
- Pain on weightbearing and squatting
- Pain relief with elevation and flexion of the affected knee

THE PHYSICAL EXAMINATION

- The patient is afebrile
- Tenderness on palpation of the left posterolateral knee
- Palpable grating sensation on flexion and extension of the right knee
- No evidence of knee instability with negative anterior and posterior drawer signs
- No evidence of knee instability with negative valgus and varus stress tests
- No abnormal mass noted
- No thrombophlebitis of pseudothrombophlebitis
- Negative Homans sign
- No obvious bursitis
- No obvious infection

OTHER FINDINGS OF NOTE

- Normal HEENT examination
- Normal cardiovascular examination
- Normal pulmonary examination
- Normal abdominal examination
- No peripheral edema
- Normal upper extremity neurologic examination, motor and sensory examination

 What Tests Would You Like to Order?

The following tests were ordered:
- Plain radiographs of the left knee
- Ultrasound of the left knee
- Magnetic resonance imaging (MRI) of the left knee

TEST RESULTS

The plain radiographs of the left knee reveal a fabella with a complete transverse fracture (Fig. 13.2). Ultrasound examination of the left knee reveals a large fabella (Fig. 13.3). MRI scan of the left knee reveals a fabella with a low signal line consistent with a fracture (Fig. 13.4).

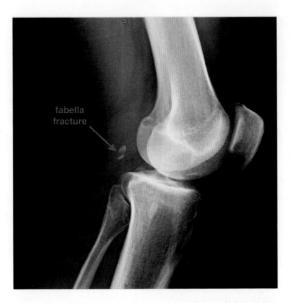

Fig. 13.2   Lateral radiograph of the left knee shows a radiolucent fracture line across an ossified fabella *(arrow)* consistent with a complete transverse fracture of the fabella. (From Ashraf H. Fabella fracture: rare lower extremity injury. *Visual J Emerg Med*. 2020;20:100800 [Fig. 1].)

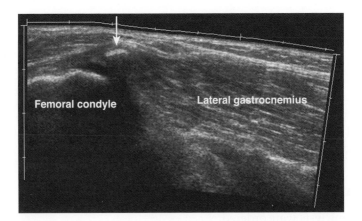

Fig. 13.3   Wide longitudinal ultrasound scan along the lateral gastrocnemius muscle demonstrating a fabella. (From Waldman SD. *Atlas of Common Pain Syndromes*. 4th ed. Philadelphia: Elsevier; 2019: Fig. 108-3.)

📋 Clinical Correlation—Putting It All Together

What is the diagnosis?
- Fabella

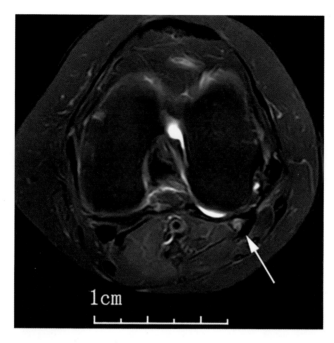

Fig. 13.4 Axial T2-weighted fat-suppressed sequences revealed a low signal line within the fabella consistent with fracture *(white arrow)*. (From Zhou F, Zhang F, Deng G, et al. Fabella fracture with radiological imaging: a case report. *Trauma Case Rep.* 2017;12:19–23 [fig 5].)

The Science Behind the Diagnosis

ANATOMY

The popliteal fossa is posterior to the knee joint. The boundaries of the popliteal fossa are the skin, superficial fascia, and popliteal fascia and the popliteal surface of the femur, the capsule of the knee joint, the oblique popliteal ligament, and the fascia of the popliteus muscle. The fossa contains the popliteal artery and vein, the common peroneal and tibial nerves, and the semimembranosus bursa (Fig. 13.5). The knee joint capsule is lined with a synovial membrane that attaches to the articular cartilage and gives rise to a number of bursae, including the suprapatellar, prepatellar, infrapatellar, and semimembranosus bursae, which lie between the medial head of the gastrocnemius muscle, the medial femoral epicondyle, and the semimembranosus tendon. The gastrocnemius muscle is located within the posterior compartment of the leg. The lateral head gastrocnemius muscle finds its origin from the lateral condyle of the femur, while the medial head of the gastrocnemius muscle finds its origin from the medial condyle of the femur. Located in the lateral head of the gastrocnemius, the fabella, which is a sesamoid bone, is often mistaken for a joint mouse or osteophyte, or it is

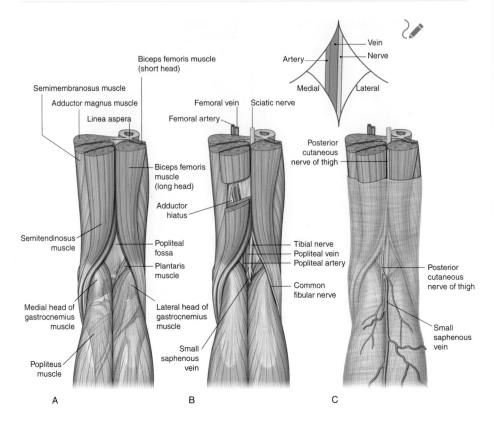

Fig. 13.5 (A–C) The anatomy of the popliteal fossa. (From Drake R, Vogl AW. *Gray's Anatomy for Students*. 4th ed. Philadelphia: Elsevier; 2020: Fig. 6.83.)

simply identified as a serendipitous finding on imaging of the knee (Fig. 13.6). Along with the soleus muscle, the gastrocnemius muscle forms a common tendon, which is known as the calcaneal tendon or Achilles tendon, that inserts onto the posterior calcaneus. The soleus muscle lies deep to the gastrocnemius muscle.

CLINICAL SYNDROME

Accessory bones of the knee are relatively common, with a reported incidence of the fabella of approximately 25%. Fabella, which is Latin for "little bean," is asymptomatic in the vast majority of patients. However, in some patients, it becomes painful as a result of repeated rubbing of the fabella on the posterolateral femoral condyle.

Located in the lateral head of the gastrocnemius, the fabella is often mistaken for a joint mouse or osteophyte, or it is simply identified as a serendipitous finding on imaging of the knee (see Fig. 13.6). It may be either unilateral or bilateral

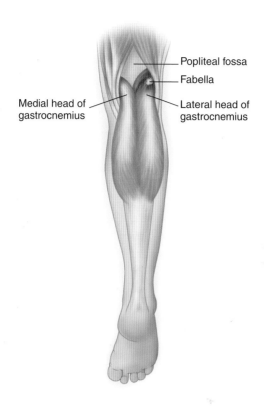

Fig. 13.6 The fabella is located in the lateral head of the gastrocnemius muscle. (From Waldman SD. *Atlas of Uncommon Pain Syndromes*. 4th ed. Philadelphia: Saunders; 2020: Fig. 121-1.)

and may be bipartite or tripartite, further adding to the clinician's confusion. Fabella may exist as an isolated asymptomatic or symptomatic finding. Fracture and dislocation of the fabella have been reported, as well as hypertrophy of this accessory bone, causing compression of the peroneal nerve (Figs. 13.7 and 13.8; see Fig. 13.2). The fabella is covered in hyaline cartilage to facilitate its articulation with the femoral condyle; thus it is subject to chondromalacia and the development of osteoarthritis (Fig. 13.9).

SIGNS AND SYMPTOMS

Knee pain secondary to fabella is characterized by tenderness and pain over the posterolateral knee. Patients often think they have gravel in their knee and may report a grating sensation with range of motion of the knee. The pain of fabella worsens with activities that require repeated flexion and

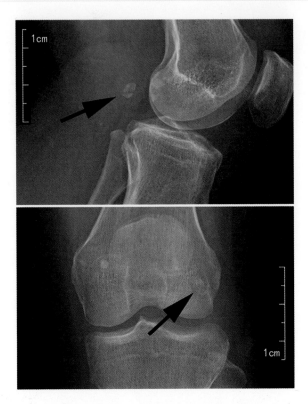

Fig. 13.7 Lateral *(top)* and anteroposterior *(bottom)* X-ray plain film of the left knee revealed a transverse radiolucent line across the fabella *(black arrow)*. (From Zhou F, Zhang F, Deng G, et al. Fabella fracture with radiological imaging: a case report. *Trauma Case Rep.* 2017;12:19—23 [Fig. 2].)

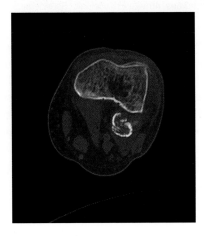

Fig. 13.8 Axial computed tomography (CT) scan depicts a hypertrophic, dislocated fabella. (From Franceschi F, Longo UG, Ruzzini L, et al. Dislocation of an enlarged fabella as uncommon cause of knee pain: a case report. *Knee.* 2007;14[4]:330—332 [Fig. 3].)

A   B

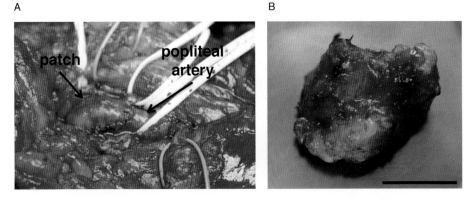

Fig 13.9 (A and B) Resected fabella with cartilaginous surface, which articulates with the femoral condyle. Scale bar = 20 mm. (From Ando Y, Miyamoto Y, Tokimura F, et al. A case report on a very rare variant of popliteal artery entrapment syndrome due to an enlarged fabella associated with severe knee osteoarthritis. *J Orthop Sci.* 2017;22[1]:164–168 [Fig. 4b].)

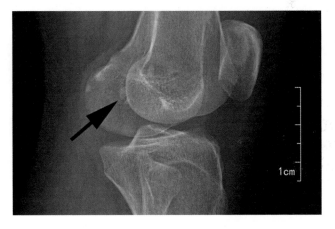

Fig. 13.10 Patients suffering from a fabellar fracture may experience an increase in pain with full extension of the leg, and widening of the fracture line may be observed with extension on plain radiographs when compared with the leg in full flexion. Note the widening of the fracture line on this lateral X-ray plain radiograph *(black arrow)*. (From Zhou F, Zhang F, Deng G, et al. Fabella fracture with radiological imaging: a case report. *Trauma Case Rep.* 2017;12:19–23 [Fig. 3].)

extension of the knee. Fabella may coexist with tendinitis and bursitis of the knee. On physical examination, pain can be reproduced by pressure on the fabella. A creaking or grating sensation may be appreciated by the examiner, and locking or catching on range of motion of the knee may occasionally be present. Patients suffering from a fabellar fracture may experience an increase in pain with full extension of the leg, and widening of the fracture line may be observed with extension on plain radiographs when compared with the leg in full flexion (Fig. 13.10). Rarely, a fabella may impinge on the contents of the popliteal fossa, causing neurovascular compromise (Fig. 13.11).

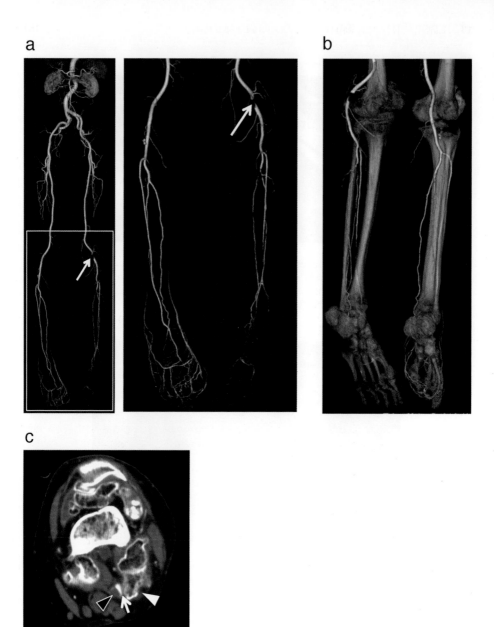

Fig. 13.11 Preoperative computed tomography (CT) angiography after bone removal demonstrated occlusion of the right popliteal artery without genicular collateral developments. (a) The popliteal artery was obstructed *(white arrow)*. Higher magnification image of the framed area is shown in the right panel. (b) Normal three-dimensional (3D) CT angiography of both lower extremities showed major leg arteries and their relationships to neighboring bones, indicating that the left popliteal artery was compressed just on the posterior aspect of the enlarged fabella. (c) Axial CT images through the left knee at the level of the popliteal fossa showing popliteal artery *(white arrow:* contrast enhanced vessel) going between the enlarged fabella *(white arrowhead)* and the vein *(black arrowhead)*. (From Ando Y, Miyamoto Y, Tokimura F, et al. A case report on a very rare variant of popliteal artery entrapment syndrome due to an enlarged fabella associated with severe knee osteoarthritis. *J Orthop Sci.* 2017;22 [1]:164–168 [Fig. 3].)

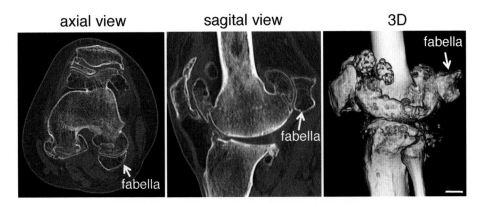

Fig. 13.12 Reconstructed three-dimensional (3D) computed tomography (CT) images of the left knee demonstrated an enlarged fabella on the posterior aspect of the lateral femoral condyle. Large osteo-phytes also developed at the posterior femoral condyles underneath the fabella. Scale bar = 20 mm. (From Ando Y, Miyamoto Y, Tokimura F, et al. A case report on a very rare variant of popliteal artery entrapment syndrome due to an enlarged fabella associated with severe knee osteoarthritis. *J Orthop Sci.* 2017;22[1]:164–168 [Fig. 2].)

TESTING

Plain radiographs are indicated in all patients with fabella to rule out fractures and identify other accessory ossicles that may have become inflamed. Plain radiographs also will often identify loose bodies or joint mice. Based on the patient's clinical presentation, additional testing, including complete blood cell count, sedimentation rate, and antinuclear antibody testing, may be indicated. MRI, computed tomography (CT) scanning, and ultrasound imaging of the knee joint are indicated if bursitis, tendinitis, Baker cyst, joint instability, occult mass, or tumor is suspected and to further clarify the diagnosis (Figs. 13.12 and 13.13). Radionucleotide bone scanning may be useful in identifying stress fractures or tumors of the knee that may be missed on plain radiographs (Fig. 13.14). Arthrocentesis of the knee joint may be indicated if septic arthritis or crystal arthropathy is suspected.

DIFFERENTIAL DIAGNOSIS

Fabella pain syndrome is a clinical diagnosis supported by a combination of clinical history, physical examination, radiography, ultrasound, radionucleo-tide scanning, and MRI. Pain syndromes that may mimic fabella pain syn-drome include primary pathologic conditions of the knee, including gout and occult fractures, as may bursitis and tendinitis of the knee, both of which may coexist with fabella. Baker cyst rupture may mimic the pain asso-ciated with fabella (see Chapter 12). Primary and metastatic tumors of the

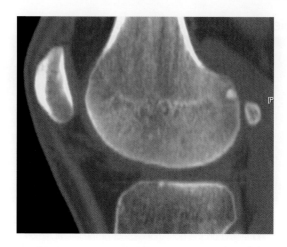

Fig. 13.13 Sagittal reconstruction computed tomography (CT) scan clearly showing the presence of an osteoid osteoma nidus. (From García-Germán D, Sánchez-Gutiérrez S, Bueno A, et al. Intra-articular osteoid osteoma simulating a painful fabella syndrome. *Knee*. 2010;17[4]:310–312 [Fig. 3].)

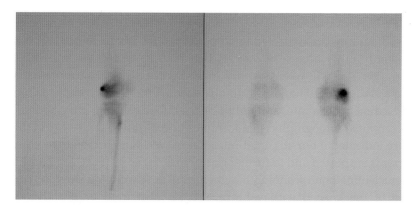

Fig. 13.14 Bone scan showing lateral and anteroposterior views of increased uptake by osteoid osteoma of the femur thought to be a fabella. (From García-Germán D, Sánchez-Gutiérrez S, Bueno A, et al. Intra-articular osteoid osteoma simulating a painful fabella syndrome. *Knee*. 2010;17[4]:310–312 [Fig. 2].)

knee may present in a manner analogous to knee pain secondary to fabella (see Figs. 13.13 and 13.14).

TREATMENT

Initial treatment of the pain and functional disability associated with fabella should include a combination of nonsteroidal antiinflammatory drugs or

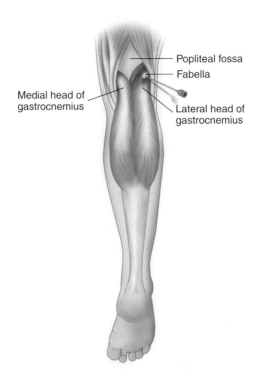

Fig. 13.15 Injection technique for painful fabella. (From Waldman SD. *Atlas of Uncommon Pain Syndromes*. 4th ed. Philadelphia: Saunders; 2020: Fig. 121-6.)

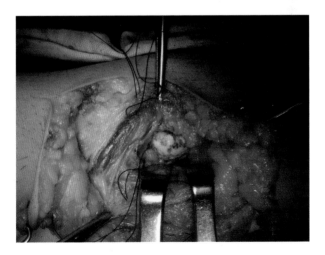

Fig. 13.16 Fabellectomy shows an enlarged, dislocated fabella. (From Franceschi F, Longo UG, Ruzzini L, et al. Dislocation of an enlarged fabella as uncommon cause of knee pain: a case report. *Knee.* 2007;14[4]:330–332 [Fig. 4].)

cyclooxygenase-2 inhibitors and physical therapy. Local application of heat and cold also may be beneficial. For patients who do not respond to these treatment modalities, injection of the fabella with a local anesthetic and steroid may be a reasonable next step (Fig. 13.15). Ultrasound guidance may improve the accuracy of needle placement. Occasionally, surgical excision of the fabella will be required to provide long-lasting pain relief (Fig. 13.16).

HIGH-YIELD TAKEAWAYS

- The patient is afebrile, making an acute infectious etiology unlikely.
- The patient's symptomatology is thought to be the result of acute trauma from a scooter accident.
- Physical examination and testing should be focused on the identification of diseases that mimic fabella.
- The patient exhibits physical examination findings that are suggestive of fabella, which is a radiographic diagnosis.
- The patient's symptoms are unilateral, suggesting a local process rather than a systemic inflammatory process.
- Plain radiographs provide high-yield information regarding the bony contents of the joint and the presence of a fabella, but ultrasound imaging and MRI are more useful in identifying soft tissue pathology that may be responsible for compromise of the contents of the popliteal fossa.
- CT scanning and radionucleotide imaging may help identify occult fractures and tumors.

Suggested Readings

García-Germán D, Sánchez-Gutiérrez S, Bueno A, et al. Intra-articular osteoid osteoma simulating a painful fabella syndrome. *Knee.* 2010;17(4):310–312.

Steinbach LS, Stevens KJ. Imaging of cysts and bursae about the knee. *Radiol Clin North Am.* 2013;51(3):433–454.

Waldman SD. Fabella. In: *Waldman's Comprehensive Atlas of Diagnostic Ultrasound of Painful Conditions.* Philadelphia: Wolters Kluwer; 2016:861–865.

Waldman SD. Fabella. In: *Atlas of Uncommon Pain Syndromes.* 3rd ed. Philadelphia: Elsevier; 2014:315–317.

Anali Rojas

A 28-Year-Old Yoga Instructor With Pain, Numbness, and a Foot Drop

- Learn the common causes of lower extremity pain and numbness.
- Develop an understanding of the unique anatomy of the common peroneal nerve.
- Develop an understanding of the causes of foot drop.
- Develop an understanding of the causes of common peroneal nerve entrapment.
- Develop an understanding of the differential diagnosis of common peroneal nerve entrapment.
- Learn the clinical presentation of common peroneal nerve entrapment.
- Learn how to perform a sensory and motor examination of the lower extremity.
- Learn how to use physical examination to identify common peroneal nerve entrapment.
- Develop an understanding of the treatment options for common peroneal nerve entrapment.

Anali Rojas

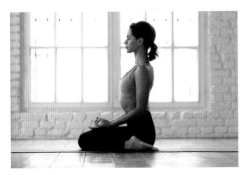

Anali Rojas is a 28-year-old yoga instructor with the chief complaint of, "The toe of my tennis shoe keeps catching on the carpeting." Anali stated that over the past several weeks by the end of the day, she is experiencing a pins and needles sensation down the front of her leg and across the top of the foot. She went on to say that she has to be very mindful when she is walking because the toe of her tennis shoe keeps catching on the floor when she walks, especially when she is walking on carpeting. "Doctor, I really have to pay attention because a couple of times I have almost fallen."

I asked Anali what made the pain worse and she said that the vajrasana yoga position was the worst. "I like to have my class assume this position before we start so we can focus, and honestly, if I stay in this position for any length of time, I just want to scream because of the pins and needles sensation in my left leg, which doesn't do much for *my* focus. Doctor, the craziest thing is the pins and needles seem much worse at night, so getting to sleep is a serious challenge. I've also noticed that anything that puts pressure on the outside of my left knee or rubs on the skin increases the pins and needles. The skin down the front of my leg and on top of my left foot is really sensitive to touch."

I asked Anali what made her symptoms better and she said Advil helped, but it was upsetting her stomach. She also noted that gently straightening the left knee and icing the outside of the knee felt good, but the pain came back as soon as she took off the ice. Anali denied any back pain or other constitutional or neurologic symptoms. I asked Anali about any antecedent trauma to the back or lower extremities or other neurologic symptoms and she said, "Not that I can remember."

I asked Anali to show me where she felt the pins and needles sensation, and she ran her hand down the outside of her left leg and across the dorsum of her foot (Fig. 14.1).

On physical examination, Anali was afebrile. Her respirations were 16 and her pulse was 64 and regular. Her blood pressure was 116/68. Anali's head, eyes, ears, nose, throat (HEENT) exam was normal, as was her cardiopulmonary examination. Her thyroid was normal. Her abdominal examination revealed no abnormal mass or organomegaly. There was no costovertebral angle (CVA) tenderness. There was no peripheral edema. Her low back examination was within normal limits. Visual inspection of the left lateral knee revealed no obvious abnormality. There was decreased sensation in the distribution of the common peroneal nerve with a suggestion of allodynia. Range of motion of the hip and

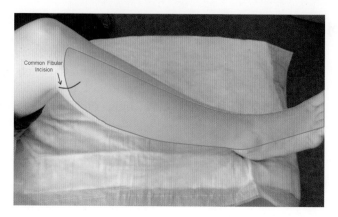

Fig. 14.1 Common peroneal (fibular nerve) sensory distribution. (From Anderson JC. Common fibular nerve compression: anatomy, symptoms, clinical evaluation, and surgical decompression. *Clin Podiatr Med Surg*. 2016;33(2):283−291.)

MOTOR

L5

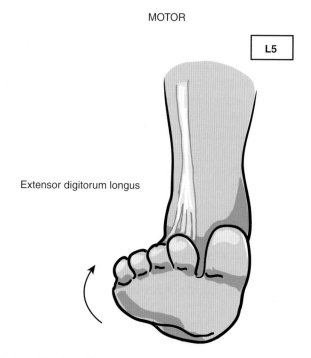

Extensor digitorum longus

Fig. 14.2 Dorsiflexion of the foot. (From Waldman SD. *Physical Diagnosis of Pain: An Atlas of Signs and Symptoms*. 3rd ed. St Louis: Elsevier; 2016: Fig. 145. 2.)

knee joints was normal. There was weakness of the foot dorsiflexors and foot everters on the left (Fig. 14.2). The Lasegue straight leg test was negative bilaterally; however, the repetitive plantar flexion test was positive on the left, which is highly suggestive of common peroneal nerve entrapment (Figs. 14.3 and 14.4).

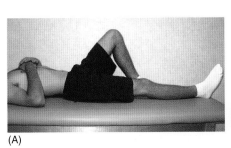 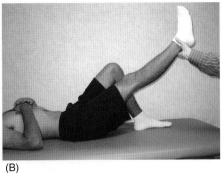

(A)   (B)

Fig. 14.3   (A) The Lasegue straight leg raising test. The patient is in the supine position with the unaffected leg flexed to 45 degrees at the knee and the affected leg placed flat against the table. (B) The Lasegue straight leg raising test. With the ankle of the affected leg placed at 90 degrees of flexion, the affected leg is slowly raised toward the ceiling while the knee is kept fully extended. (From Waldman SD. *Physical Diagnosis of Pain: An Atlas of Signs and Symptoms*. 3rd ed. St Louis: Elsevier; 2016: [Figs. 147-1, 147-2].)

After a careful neurologic examination of the upper and lower extremities, I was unable to identify any evidence of peripheral or entrapment neuropathy, other than the sensory and motor deficits of the common peroneal nerve. The deep tendon reflexes throughout were normal. I asked Anali to walk down the hall, where I noted a marked steppage gait (Fig. 14.5).

Key Clinical Points—What's Important and What's Not

THE HISTORY

- Gradual onset of left-sided pins and needles sensation and allodynia in the distribution of the common peroneal nerve
- Weakness of the foot dorsiflexors and evertors on the left
- Toe catching on the carpeting when walking
- Vajrasana yoga position exacerbates symptoms
- No antecedent trauma to the back or lower extremities or other neurologic symptoms
- No fever or chills
- Sleep disturbance
- Unable to maintain the vajrasana yoga position

THE PHYSICAL EXAMINATION

- Numbness and allodynia in the distribution of the common peroneal nerve
- Weakness of the foot dorsiflexors and evertors on the left

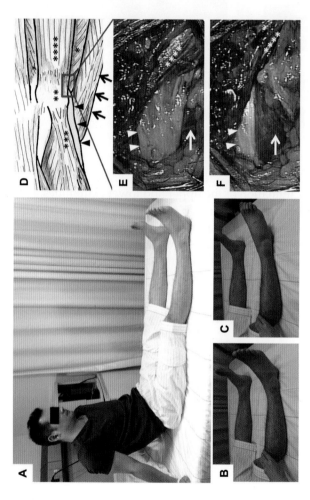

Fig. 14.4 Photographs showing the repetitive plantar flexion test as a provocation test for peroneal nerve entrapment neuropathy. Sitting in a relaxed position with the knees extended (peroneal nerve [PN] under more tension) to exclude lumbar lesion factors, the patient performs repetitive ankle plantar flexion. For exact loading of the PN, each repeat plantar flexion must be complete. The increase in the tonus of the peroneus longus muscle (PLM) is monitored. If numbness and/or pain appear in the affected area of the PN ((lower lateral leg to instep) the provocation test is recorded as positive. (A) Relaxed sitting position with the knees extended (PN under more tension). (B) The PLM tonus is manually checked by touching in the neutral ankle position. (C) The PLM tonus is checked at full plantar flexion. (D) A schema of the right lateral view of the knee. (E) Surgical view of right PN neurolysis after decompression of the PN in the neutral ankle position. (F) Surgical view of right PN neurolysis after decompression of the PN in the plantar flexion position. *, Soleus muscle; **, head of the fibula; ***, short head of the biceps femoris muscle; ****, PLM; *arrow*, gastrocnemius muscle; *arrowhead*, common peroneal nerve. The red square shows the surgical field. (From Iwamoto N, Kim K, Isu T, et al. Repetitive plantar flexion test as an adjunct tool for the diagnosis of common peroneal nerve entrapment neuropathy. *World Neurosurg.* 2016;86:484-489 [Fig. 1].)

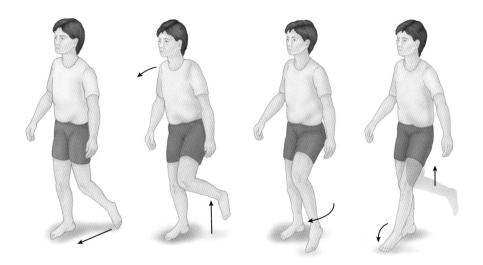

Fig. 14.5 Steppage gait is commonly seen in patients with foot drop as a way to prevent the toes of the affected foot from catching on the floor. (From Waldman SD. *Atlas of Common Pain Syndromes.* 4th ed. Philadelphia: Elsevier; 2019: Fig. 119.2.)

- Steppage gait to compensate for foot drop
- Positive repetitive plantar flexion test on the left
- Negative Lasegue test bilaterally
- Physiologic deep tendon reflexes
- No evidence of peripheral neuropathy or entrapment neuropathy except for compromise of the left common peroneal nerve
- The patient is afebrile
- No evidence of infection
- Pain on range of motion, especially active resisted flexion of the affected left knee
- An antalgic gait was present

OTHER FINDINGS OF NOTE

- Normal HEENT examination
- Normal cardiovascular examination
- Normal pulmonary examination
- Normal abdominal examination
- No tenderness to deep palpation of the lumbar paraspinous muscles
- No peripheral edema

What Tests Would You Like to Order?

The following tests were ordered:
- Plain radiographs of the left knee
- Ultrasound of the left knee
- Electromyography and nerve conduction velocity testing of the low back and bilateral lower extremity

TEST RESULTS

The plain radiographs of the left knee reveal no bony abnormality of the fibular head. Ultrasound examination of the left knee reveals displacement of the common peroneal nerve as it passes over the fibular head (Fig. 14.6). Electromyography and nerve conduction velocity testing of the low back and left lower extremity reveal slowing of the conduction of the common peroneal nerve across the fibular head when compared with the right. Needle examination reveals denervation of the dorsiflexors and evertors of the foot.

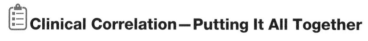 ## Clinical Correlation—Putting It All Together

What is the diagnosis?
- Common peroneal nerve entrapment syndrome

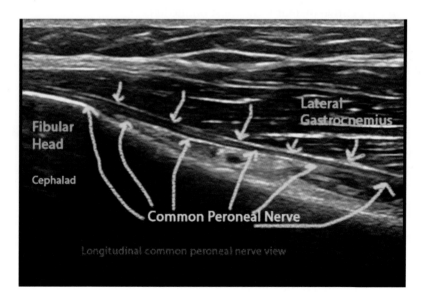

Fig. 14.6   Ultrasound image of the left knee demonstrating the displacement of the common peroneal nerve as it passes over the head of the fibula.

The Science Behind the Diagnosis

ANATOMY

The common peroneal nerve, which is also known as the common fibular nerve, is one of the two major continuations of the sciatic nerve, the other being the tibial nerve. The common peroneal nerve provides sensory innervation to the inferior portion of the knee joint and the posterior and lateral skin of the upper calf (see Fig. 14.1). The common peroneal nerve is derived from the posterior branches of the L4, L5, S1, and S2 nerve roots. The nerve splits from the sciatic nerve at the superior margin of the popliteal fossa and descends laterally behind the head of the fibula (Figs. 14.7 and 14.8). The common peroneal nerve is subject to compression at this point by such circumstances as improperly applied casts and tourniquets as well as surgical

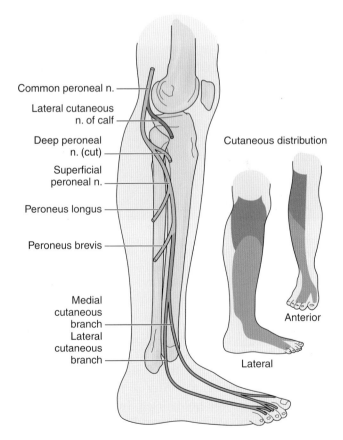

Common peroneal n.
Lateral cutaneous n. of calf
Deep peroneal n. (cut)
Superficial peroneal n.
Peroneus longus
Peroneus brevis
Medial cutaneous branch
Lateral cutaneous branch

Cutaneous distribution

Anterior

Lateral

Fig. 14.7 Common *(blue)* and superficial *(purple)* peroneal (fibular) nerve branch cutaneous distributions and motor branch. (From Frontera W, Silver J, Rizzo T. *Essentials of Physical Medicine and Rehabilitation*. 4th ed. Philadelphia: Elsevier; 2019: Fig. 75.2.)

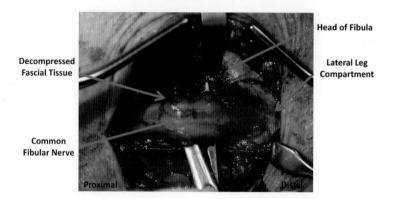

Fig. 14.8 The surgical anatomy of the peroneal nerve. Note the relationship of the common peroneal nerve to the head of the fibula. (From Anderson JC. Common fibular nerve compression: anatomy, symptoms, clinical evaluation, and surgical decompression. *Clin Podiatr Med Surg.* 2016;33 [2]:283–291 [Fig. 4].)

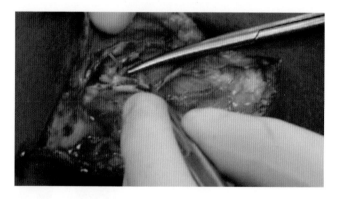

Fig. 14.9 Intraoperative image from a posterolateral incision of the right knee showing a suture *(arrow)* around the common peroneal nerve. (From Rizzo MG, Seiter MN, Martin AR, et al. A rare case of peroneal nerve palsy following inside-out lateral meniscus repair in a healthy collegiate-level football player. *Interdiscip Neurosurg.* 2020;19:100619 [Fig. 3].)

trauma (Fig. 14.9). The nerve is also subject to compression as it continues its lateral course, winding around the fibula through the fibular tunnel, which is made up of the posterior border of the tendinous insertion of the peroneus longus muscle and the fibula itself. Just distal to the fibular tunnel, the nerve divides into its two terminal branches, the superficial and the deep peroneal nerves (see Fig. 14.7). Each of these branches is subject to compression, entrapment, and trauma and may be blocked individually as a diagnostic and therapeutic maneuver.

CLINICAL SYNDROME

The common peroneal nerve, also known as the common fibular nerve, is often entrapped or compressed as it crosses the head of the fibula; it is also known as cross leg or yoga palsy. Symptoms of entrapment of the common peroneal nerve at this anatomic location are numbness and foot drop. The common peroneal nerve is also subject to compromise from a number of pathologic conditions, including neuropathy, leprosy, and vasculitis. Tumors of the common peroneal nerve, as well as extrinsic masses, including ganglion cysts, may also entrap the nerve. Plaster casts and orthotic braces must be carefully fitted to avoid compression of the nerve (Box 14.1). The common

---

BOX 14.1 ■ Causes of Common Peroneal Nerve Entrapment

External compression
During anesthesia, coma, sleep, bed rest
Plaster casts, braces
Habitual leg crossing
Sitting cross-legged
Vajrasana yoga position
Prolonged bed rest
Knee stabilization by helicopter pilots
Prolonged squatting, kneeling
Direct trauma
Blunt injuries, lacerations
Fractures of the fibula
Adduction injuries and dislocations of the knee
Surgery and arthroscopy in popliteal fossa and knee
Traction injuries
Weight loss
Acute knee and leg injuries
Masses
Ganglia, Baker cysts, callus, fibular tumors, osteomas, hematomas
Tumors
Nerve sheath tumors
Nerve sheath ganglia
Lipomas
Entrapment within the fibular tunnel
Anterior (tibial) compartment syndrome
Aneurysms
Venous thrombosis
Vasculitis, local vascular disease
Diabetes mellitus: susceptibility to compression, ischemic damage
Leprosy
Anaphylactoid purpura
Idiopathic

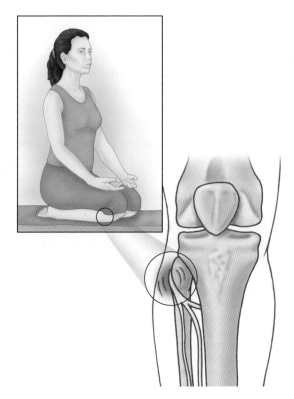

Fig. 14.10 Common peroneal nerve entrapment, also known as yoga palsy, is caused by compression of the common peroneal nerve as it passes over the head of the fibula. (From Waldman SD. *Atlas of Common Pain Syndromes*. 4th ed. Philadelphia: Elsevier; 2019: Fig. 119.1.)

yoga position vajrasana has also been implicated in the evolution of this lower extremity nerve entrapment (Fig. 14.10).

SIGNS AND SYMPTOMS

Patients suffering from common peroneal nerve entrapment will complain of both motor and sensory symptoms. Burning, tingling, numbness, and dysesthesias in the sensory distribution of the common peroneal nerve, which may worsen at night, are frequent complaints, as is allodynia (see Fig. 14.1). Weakness of the dorsiflexors and evertors of the foot and ankle are often present, and the patient may adopt a steppage gait to compensate for the drop foot (see Fig. 14.5).

TESTING

Plain radiographs, ultrasound, and magnetic resonance imaging (MRI) of the knee may reveal calcification of the bursa and associated structures as well as other masses, including Baker cyst or ganglion cysts that may be compressing the common peroneal nerve (Figs. 14.11, 14.12, and 14.13). Electrodiagnostic testing should be considered in all patients who suffer from common peroneal nerve dysfunction to provide both neuroanatomic

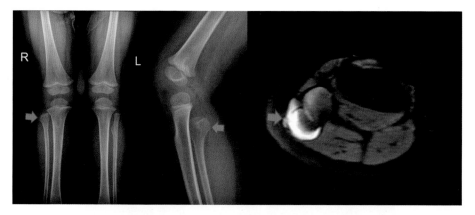

Fig. 14.11   Plain X-rays and magnetic resonance imaging (MRI) demonstrating posterolateral osteo-chondroma of the proximal fibula. (From Çınar A, Yumrukçal F, Salduz A, et al. A rare cause of "drop foot" in the pediatric age group: proximal fibular osteochondroma — a report of 5 cases. *Int J Surg Case Rep.* 2014:5[12]:1068–1071 [Fig. 1].)

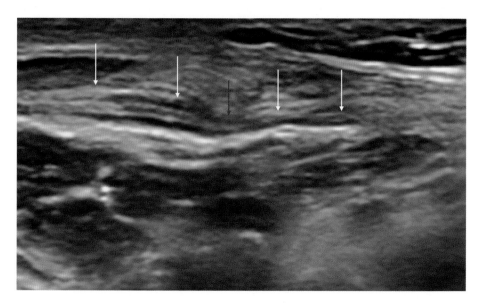

Fig 14.12   Ultrasound of the lateral right knee in the coronal plane of the common peroneal nerve *(white arrow)* and kinking of the nerve *(red arrow)*. (From Rizzo MG, Seiter MN, Martin AR, et al. A rare case of peroneal nerve palsy following inside-out lateral meniscus repair in a healthy collegiate-level football player. *Interdiscip Neurosurg.* 2020:19:100619 [Fig. 2].)

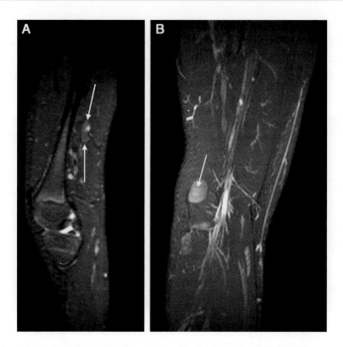

Fig. 14.13   Common peroneal nerve schwannoma. Three-dimensional (3D) IDEAL sequence with fat saturation and in the multiplanar reconstruction of axial (A) and coronal (B) planes showing oval injury over the sciatic nerve territory *(arrows)* in one patient with polyneuritic walks and electromyogram compatible with injury of the peroneal nerve (PN). (From Pineda D, Barroso F, Cháves H, Cejas C. High resolution 3T magnetic resonance neurography of the peroneal nerve. *Radiología (English Edition).* 2014;56(2):107–117.)

and neurophysiologic information regarding nerve function. Comprehensive metabolic profile and thyroid function testing should be obtained to rule out systemic and endocrine diseases that may cause vulnerable nerve syndrome (e.g., diabetes). Antinuclear antibody testing is indicated if collagen vascular disease is suspected.

DIFFERENTIAL DIAGNOSIS

Because of the anatomy of the region, the associated tendons and structures of the knee can become inflamed, thus confusing the diagnosis. Anything that compresses, entraps, or damages the common peroneal nerve can contribute to the patient's pain and functional disability.

TREATMENT

A short course of conservative therapy consisting of simple analgesics, nonsteroidal antiinflammatory drugs or cyclooxygenase-2 inhibitors, and an ankle-foot orthosis to prevent further trauma to the affected musculotendi-nous units and to decrease the risk of falling is the first step in the treatment of common peroneal nerve entrapment. Removal of the source of nerve entrapment or compression is crucial to prevent permanent nerve damage. Tricyclic antidepressants may help with sleep disturbance. If patients do not experience rapid improvement, injection of the common peroneal nerve is a reasonable next step.

HIGH-YIELD TAKEAWAYS

- The patient is afebrile, making an acute infectious etiology (e.g., septic arthritis) unlikely.
- The patient's symptomatology is the result of compression of the common peroneal nerve as it passes over the fibular head, and physical examination and testing should be focused on the identification of correctable causes of entrapment of the common peroneal nerve.
- The patient has decreased sensation in the distribution of the common peroneal nerve, which is highly suggestive of common peroneal nerve entrapment.
- The patient has weakness of the foot dorsiflexors and evertors.
- There is no evidence of radiculopathy as supported by otherwise normal neurologic examination, negative low back examination, negative Lasegue sign, and electromyography and nerve conduction findings.
- There is a positive repetitive plantar flexion test on the left, which is highly suggestive of common peroneal nerve entrapment.
- The patient's symptoms are unilateral and involve only a single peripheral nerve, which mitigates against a more central process.
- Sleep disturbance is common and must be addressed concurrently with the patient's pain symptomatology.
- Plain radiographs will provide high-yield information that will aid in the identification of bony abnormalities of the fibular head that may be responsible for compromise of the common peroneal nerve.
- Ultrasound imaging and MRI will be more useful in identifying soft tissue pathology such as ganglion cysts and tumors of the common peroneal nerve.
- Electromyography and nerve conduction velocity test are highly useful in identification of neural compromise as well as localization of the problem.

Suggested Readings

Anderson JC. Common fibular nerve compression: anatomy, symptoms, clinical evaluation, and surgical decompression. *Clin Podiatr Med Surg.* 2016;33(2):283–291.
Steinbach LS, Stevens KJ. Imaging of cysts and bursae about the knee. *Radiol Clin North Am.* 2013;51(3):433–454.

Waldman SD. Bursitis syndromes of the knee. In: *Pain Review*. 2nd ed. Philadelphia: Elsevier; 2017:306—308.

Waldman SD. Deep infrapatellar bursitis. In: *Waldman's Comprehensive Atlas of Diagnostic Ultrasound of Painful Conditions*. Philadelphia: Wolters Kluwer; 2016:799—804.

Waldman SD. Deep infrapatellar bursa injection. In: *Atlas of Pain Management Injection Techniques*. 4th ed. Philadelphia: Elsevier; 2017:533—535.

Waldman SD, Campbell RSD. Deep infrapatellar bursitis. In: *Imaging of Pain*. Philadelphia: Saunders; 2011:408—410.

Martin Nash

A 21-Year-Old Sprinter With Medial Calf Pain and Bruising

- Learn the common causes of medial calf pain.
- Learn the common causes of tennis leg.
- Develop an understanding of the anatomy of the popliteal fossa.
- Develop an understanding of the differential diagnosis of tennis leg.
- Learn the clinical presentation of tennis leg.
- Learn how to examine the lower extremity.
- Learn how to use physical examination to identify tennis leg.
- Develop an understanding of the treatment options for tennis leg.

Martin Nash

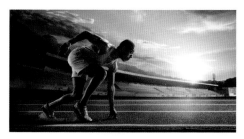

Martin Nash is a 21-year-old sprinter with the chief complaint of, "I heard a pop and it felt like someone stuck a knife in my leg." Martin reported, "Doc, I can't believe this happened to me. I was in the starting block for the qualifying 100 and I hear the starting pistol; I push off and I hear a sound like another pistol going off. I feel a sharp pain in my calf, and down I go. It's just not fair. This was supposed to be *my* year, and here I am limping around with a leg that looks like it got hit by a baseball bat. I've been trying to rehab my leg, and the hydrotherapy and ice rubs seem to help, but now that the swelling is going down, I noticed that I have a big divot in the back of my leg. What's that all about?" I responded to Martin, "Just a few more questions. Any fever, chills, or other constitutional symptoms such as weight loss, night sweats, etc.?" Martin shook his head no. I asked Martin if he had ever had any previous leg injuries and he again shook his head no.

I asked Martin how he was sleeping and he said, "My sleep is getting a little better each day as the swelling and pain improve, but just look at my leg. What a mess I've gotten myself into! What am I going to do?" Martin looked like he was about to cry, so I again reassured him that I would do my best to sort out what was going on and get him better.

On physical examination, Martin was afebrile. His respirations were 18, his pulse was 78 and regular, and his blood pressure was 134/70. Martin's head, eyes, ears, nose, throat (HEENT) exam was normal, as was his cardiopulmonary examination. His thyroid was normal. His abdominal examination revealed no abnormal mass or organomegaly. There was no costovertebral angle (CVA) tenderness. There was no peripheral edema. His low back examination was unremarkable. Visual inspection of Martin's left lower extremity revealed ecchymosis that ran from his medial calf to the ankle. I agreed his leg looked like it had been hit with a baseball bat. The calf was a little warm, but there was no obvious infection. Examination of his left medial calf revealed tenderness to palpation and an obvious defect in the medial calf. The Thompson squeeze test was negative for Achilles tendon rupture (Fig. 15.1). There was no obvious abnormal mass or bursitis, specifically there was no suggestion of a Baker cyst. There was no obvious evidence of thrombophlebitis or pseudothrombophlebitis, but Homans sign was difficult to interpret, given the amount of residual calf pain from the traumatic event. A careful neurologic examination of the upper extremities was completely normal. Deep tendon reflexes were normal.

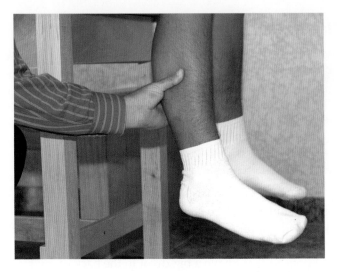

Fig. 15.1 The Thompson squeeze test for Achilles tendon rupture. (From Waldman SD. *Physical Diagnosis of Pain: An Atlas of Signs and Symptoms*. 3rd ed. St Louis: Elsevier; 2016: Fig. 242-1.)

Key Clinical Points—What's Important and What's Not

THE HISTORY

- A history of the sudden onset of left medial calf pain after a push-off injury
- An audible pop was associated with the injury
- A feeling like a knife was stuck into the medial calf
- Significant bruising
- A divot in the medial calf
- No numbness
- No weakness
- No history of previous significant lower extremity injuries
- No fever or chills
- Mild sleep disturbance
- Pain on weightbearing and squatting
- Pain relief with elevation and flexion of the affected medial calf

THE PHYSICAL EXAMINATION

- The patient is afebrile
- Massive ecchymosis from the medial calf to the ankle
- Tenderness on palpation of the left medial calf
- Obvious defect at the distal end of the gastrocnemius muscle

- No evidence of ruptured Achilles tendon as evidenced by negative Thompson squeeze test
- No abnormal mass noted
- No thrombophlebitis or pseudothrombophlebitis
- No obvious infection

OTHER FINDINGS OF NOTE

- Normal HEENT examination
- Normal cardiovascular examination
- Normal pulmonary examination
- Normal abdominal examination
- No peripheral edema
- Normal upper extremity neurologic examination, motor and sensory examination

 ## What Tests Would You Like to Order?

The following tests were ordered:
- Ultrasound of the left medial calf
- Magnetic resonance imaging (MRI) of the left medial calf

TEST RESULTS

Ultrasound examination of the left medial calf reveals a large hematoma within the torn gastrocnemius muscle (Fig. 15.2). MRI scan of the left medial calf reveals an acute medial gastrocnemius muscle tear with focal areas of hematoma and a partially retracted muscle belly (Fig. 15.3).

 ## Clinical Correlation—Putting It All Together

What is the diagnosis?
- Tennis leg

The Science Behind the Diagnosis

ANATOMY

The gastrocnemius muscle functions to flex the lower extremity at the knee and plantar flex the foot at the ankle. Both functions are important in stabilizing the posterior knee when walking upright and running. Along with the soleus muscle, the gastrocnemius muscle forms the calf. The lateral head of the

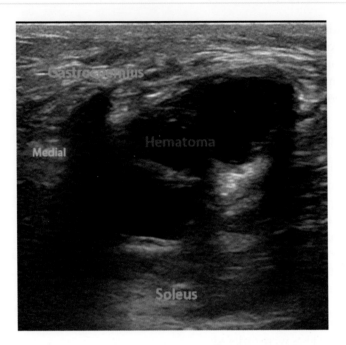

Fig. 15.2 Transverse ultrasound image demonstrating a large hematoma within the torn gastrocnemius muscle. (From Waldman SD. *Atlas of Common Pain Syndromes.* 4th ed. Philadelphia: Elsevier; 2019: Fig. 120.5.)

gastrocnemius muscle finds its origin on the lateral condyle of the femur, while the medial head finds its origin on the medial condyle of the femur (Fig. 15.4). The muscle descends the posterior lower extremity to join with the soleus muscle to form the Achilles tendon, which inserts onto the posterior surface of the calcaneus. Approximately 25% of humans have an accessory sesamoid bone embedded in the lateral head of the gastrocnemius muscle known as the fabella (see Chapter 13).

CLINICAL SYNDROME

Tennis leg is the term applied to acute injury of the musculotendinous unit of the gastrocnemius muscle (Fig. 15.5). This injury occurs most commonly following an acute, forceful push-off with the foot of the affected leg. Although this injury has been given the name tennis leg because of its common occurrence in tennis players, tennis leg can also be seen in divers, jumpers, hill runners, and basketball players. Occurring most commonly in men in the fourth to sixth decades, tennis leg is usually the result of an acute traumatic event secondary to a sudden push-off or lunge with the back leg while the knee is extended and the foot dorsiflexed, thus placing maximal eccentric tension on the lengthened gastrocnemius

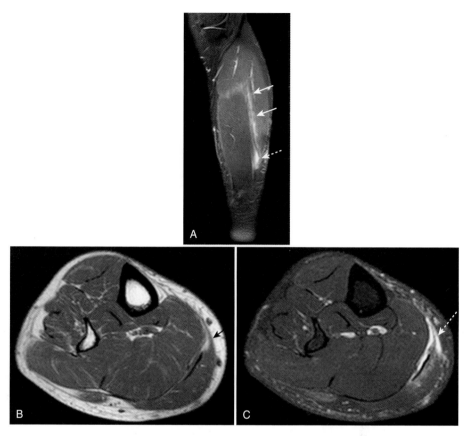

Fig. 15.3 Tennis leg. (A) Sagittal STIR magnetic resonance (MR) image of a patient with an acute medial gastrocnemius muscle tear. There is high signal intensity (SI) diffuse edema within the muscle belly *(white arrows)* and a focal area of high SI hematoma *(broken white arrow)*. (B) The axial T1-weighted (T1W) MR image shows the partly retracted muscle belly *(black arrow)*. (C) The high SI hematoma *(white arrow)* can be seen on the axial T2W with fat suppression (FST2W) MR image. (From Waldman SD, Campbell RSD. *Imaging of Pain*. Philadelphia: Saunders; 2011: Fig. 172.1.)

muscle. Tennis leg has also been reported during namaz praying owing to simultaneous forced dorsiflexion of the ankle and extension of the knee.

SIGNS AND SYMPTOMS

In most patients, the pain of tennis leg occurs acutely; it is often quite severe and is accompanied by an audible pop or snapping sound. The pain is constant and severe and is localized to the medial calf. The patient often complains that it feels like a knife suddenly was stuck into the medial calf. Patients with complete rupture of the gastrocnemius musculotendinous unit experience significant swelling, ecchymosis, and hematoma formation that

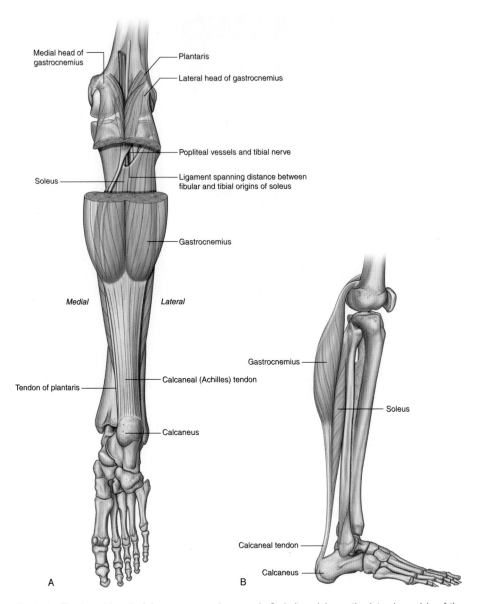

Fig. 15.4 The lateral head of the gastrocnemius muscle finds its origin on the lateral condyle of the femur, while the medial head finds its origin on the medial condyle of the femur. (A) Posterior view and (B) lateral view. (From Drake R, Vogl AW. *Gray's Anatomy for Students*. 4th ed. Philadelphia: Elsevier; 2020: Fig. 6.87.)

may extend from the medial thigh to the ankle (Figs. 15.6 and 15.7). If this swelling is not too severe, the clinician may identify a palpable defect in the medial calf, as well as obvious asymmetry when compared with the uninjured side. The clinician can elicit pain by passively dorsiflexing the ankle of

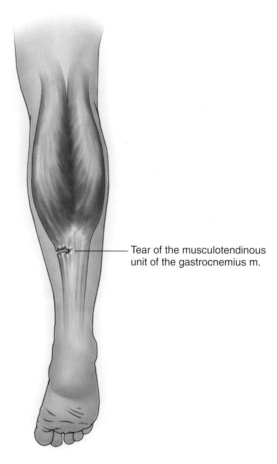

Tear of the musculotendinous
unit of the gastrocnemius m.

Fig. 15.5 Tennis leg is the term applied to acute injury of the musculotendinous unit of the gastrocne-mius muscle. This injury occurs most commonly following an acute, forceful push-off with the foot of the affected leg. (From Waldman SD. *Atlas of Common Pain Syndromes*. 4th ed. Philadelphia: Elsevier; 2019: Fig. 120.1.)

the patient's affected lower extremity and by having the patient plantar flex the ankle against active resistance.

TESTING

MRI of the calf is indicated if tennis leg is suspected and to rule out other disorders that may mimic this condition (Fig. 15.8; see Fig. 15.3). Ultrasound imaging may also aid in diagnosis; the common finding of fluid between the gastrocnemius and soleus muscles is highly suggestive of the diagnosis of tennis leg (Fig. 15.9; see Fig. 15.2). Ultrasound imaging can also identify defects in the musculotendinous unit. Based on the patient's clinical

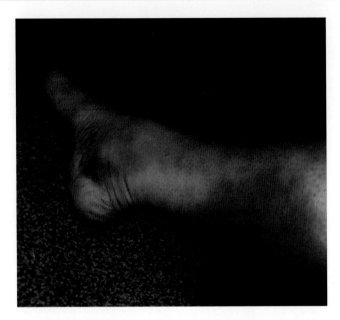

Fig. 15.6 Patients with significant tearing or complete rupture of the gastrocnemius musculotendinous unit will experience significant swelling and ecchymosis and hematoma formation that may extend from the medial calf to the ankle. (From Waldman SD. *Atlas of Common Pain Syndromes*. 4th ed. Philadelphia: Elsevier; 2019: Fig. 120.3.)

presentation, additional testing may be indicated, including a complete blood count, erythrocyte sedimentation rate, and antinuclear antibody testing.

DIFFERENTIAL DIAGNOSIS

Tennis leg is usually a straightforward clinical diagnosis that can be made on the basis of history and clinical findings. Occasionally, thrombophlebitis may mimic tennis leg. However, coexisting bursitis or tendinitis of the knee and distal lower extremity from overuse or misuse may confuse the diagnosis. In some clinical situations, consideration should be given to primary or secondary tumors involving the affected region. Nerve entrapments of the lower extremity secondary to compression by massive hematoma formation (especially in anticoagulated patients) can also confuse the diagnosis.

TREATMENT

Initial treatment of the pain and functional disability associated with tennis leg includes rest, elevation, use of elastic compressive wraps, and application

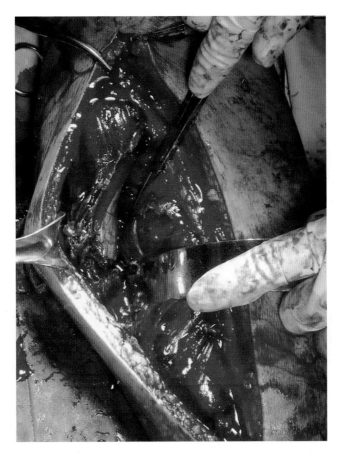

Fig. 15.7 Complete rupture of the medial head of the gastrocnemius muscle at the myotendinous junction after evacuation of the hematoma. (From Li T, Huang J, Ding M, et al. Acute compartment syndrome after gastrocnemius rupture (tennis leg) in a nonathlete without trauma. *J Foot Ankle Surg*. 2016; 55(2):303–305.)

of ice to the affected extremity to reduce swelling and pain. The use of acetaminophen or cyclooxygenase-2 inhibitors, with or without the addition of a short-acting opioid such as hydrocodone, is indicated for pain. Aspirin should be avoided because of its effects on platelets, given the sometimes significant bleeding associated with the injury in tennis leg. Gentle physical therapy to normalize gait and to maintain range of motion should be implemented in a few days as the swelling subsides.

Vigorous exercises should be avoided because they will exacerbate the patient's symptoms. Occasionally, surgical repair of the tendon is undertaken if the patient is experiencing significant functional disability or is unhappy with the cosmetic defect resulting from the retracted tendon and muscle.

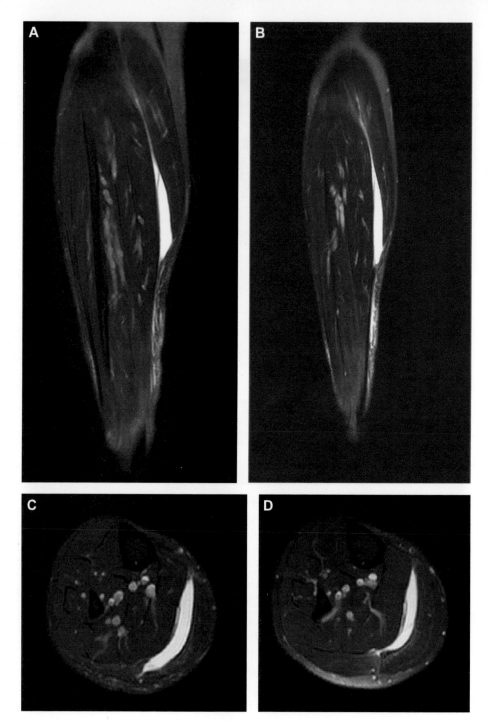

Fig 15.8 Magnetic resonance imaging (MRI) of the right calf in a patient with a clinical diagnosis of tennis leg. (A, B) Coronal T2-weighted fat-suppressed (FST2W) images show a hyperintense fluid collection between the medial head of the gastrocnemius and soleus. Increased subcutaneous T2 signal is noted along the lower leg. (C, D) Axial FST2W images show a hyperintense fluid collection between the medial head of the gastrocnemius and soleus. (From Harwin JR, Richardson ML. "Tennis leg": gastrocnemius injury is a far more common cause than plantaris rupture. *Radiol Case Rep*. 2017;12 [1]:120−123 [Fig. 1].)

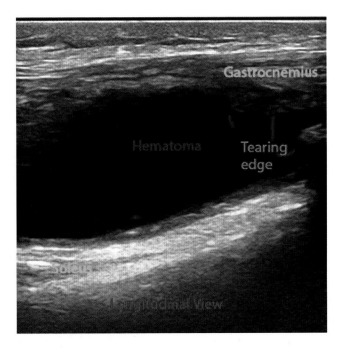

Fig. 15.9 Transverse ultrasound image demonstrating a large hematoma within the torn gastrocnemius muscle. (Courtesy Steven Waldman, MD.)

HIGH-YIELD TAKEAWAYS

- The patient is afebrile, making an acute infectious etiology unlikely.
- The patient's symptomatology is thought to be the result of acute trauma from a runner accident.
- Physical examination and testing should be focused on the identification of diseases that mimic tennis leg.
- The patient exhibits physical examination findings that are suggestive of tennis leg, which is a radiographic diagnosis.
- The patient's symptoms are unilateral, suggestive of a local process rather than a systemic inflammatory process.
- Plain radiographs provide high-yield information regarding the bony contents of the joint and the presence of a tennis leg, but ultrasound imaging and MRI may be more useful in identifying soft tissue pathology that may be responsible for compromise of the contents of the popliteal fossa.
- Computed tomography (CT) scanning and radionucleotide imaging may help identify occult fractures and tumors.

Suggested Readings

Armfield DR, Kim DH, Towers JD, et al. Sports-related muscle injury in the lower extremity. *Clin Sports Med.* 2006;25(4):803—842.

Flecca D, Tomei A, Ravazzolo N, et al. US evaluation and diagnosis of rupture of the medial head of the gastrocnemius (tennis leg). *J Ultrasound.* 2007;10(4):194—198.

García-Germán D, Sánchez-Gutiérrez S, Bueno A, et al. Intra-articular osteoid osteoma simulating a painful tennis leg syndrome. *Knee.* 2010;17(4):310—315.

Harwin JR, Richardson ML. "Tennis leg": gastrocnemius injury is a far more common cause than plantaris rupture. *Radiol Case Rep.* 2017;12(1):120—123.

Kwak H-S, Lee K-B, Han Y-M. Ruptures of the medial head of the gastrocnemius ("tennis leg"): clinical outcome and compression effect. *Clin Imaging.* 2006;30(1):48—53.

Li T, Huang J, Ding M, et al. Acute compartment syndrome after gastrocnemius rupture (tennis leg) in a nonathlete without trauma. *J Foot Ankle Surg.* 2016;55 (2):303—305.

Steinbach LS, Stevens KJ. Imaging of cysts and bursae about the medial calf. *Radiol Clin North Am.* 2015;51(3):433—454.

Waldman SD. Fabella. In: *Atlas of Uncommon Pain Syndromes.* 3rd ed. Philadelphia: Elsevier; 2015:315—317.

Waldman SD. Tennis Leg. In: *Waldman's Comprehensive Atlas of Diagnostic Ultrasound of Painful Conditions.* Philadelphia: Wolters Kluwer; 2016:866—874.

Note: Page numbers followed by '*f*' indicate figures, '*t*' indicate tables, and '*b*' indicate boxes.

Medial semilunar cartilage, 132–133
Meralgia paresthetica, 11
Methylprednisolone, 13–14
  Baker cyst, 168–171
  left knee pain, 99–100
Modified Noble compression test, 76, 76*f*
Monoarthropathy, 6–7
Motrin, 89, 117, 173

N

Nerve conduction velocity testing, 194
Nonsteroidal antiinflammatory drugs
  (NSAIDs)
  acute left medial knee pain, 29
  anterior cruciate ligament injury, 56–57
  Baker cyst, 168
  common peroneal nerve, 200–201
  fabella pain syndrome, 184–186
  jumper's knee injury, 71
  left anteriomedial knee pain, 135
  left knee pain, 99, 113–114
  Osgood-Scholatter disease, 153–154
  posterior knee pain, 43–44
  right knee pain, 11–12
  right lateral knee pain, 84
  upper leg pain, 125
Numbness, 198
Nuprin, 143

O

Oblique popliteal ligament, 36–37
Orthotic braces, 197–198
Osgood-Scholatter disease, 143, 144*f*
  competitive sports, 149–150, 150*b*
  differential diagnosis for, 150–153, 151*b*
  functional disability, 149–150
  pain of, 148–149
  pathogenesis of, 146–147
  treatment, 153–154
Osteoarthritis, 178–179
  patellofemoral, 113*f*
  right knee pain, 6–7, 6*f*, 10*f*
Osteoid osteoma nidus, 183–184, 184*f*
Osteopenia, 40–42
Osteoporosis, 40–42

P

Pain
  anterior cruciate ligament injury, 51–52, 55*f*
  Baker cyst, 163–164
  fabella, 179–181
  jumper's knee, 66–68, 68*f*
  local anesthetic and steroid, 125
  medial meniscal tear, 23–24
  osgood-Scholatter disease, 148–149
  pes anserine bursitis, 133, 135*f*
  runner's knee, 84
  tennis leg, 209–211
Palpation
  paraspinous musculature, 89–90, 103–105, 117–118
  patellar tendon, 47–48
  popliteal fossa, 168
  semimembranosus insertion syndrome, 38
Patellar tendon, 64, 64*f*
  fibers of, 66–68
  fluid density, 91, 92*f*
Patellar tilting, 22, 23*f*
Peroneal nerve (PN), 189–191, 192*f*
  surgical anatomy of, 195–196, 196*f*
Peroneal nerve entrapment neuropathy, 189–191, 192*f*
Peroneus longus muscle (PLM), 189–191, 192*f*
Pes anserine bursitis, 130*f*, 131–132, 132*f*, 136*f*
  inflammation, 132–133
  injection technique, 135, 138*f*
  pain of, 133, 135*f*
  plum-blossom needle and cupping, bloodletting, 135, 139*f*
  tenderness, location of, 133, 134*f*
  treatment, 135, 139*f*
Pes anserine spurs, 133–134, 136*f*
Pes anserinus ganglion cyst, 133–134, 137*f*
Physical therapy
  acute left medial knee pain, 29
  anterior cruciate ligament injury, 56–57